Hiit

Fastest Way to Burn Fat and Lose Weight

(Effective High Intensity Interval Training Workouts, Exercises, and Routines- Hiit Workouts)

Elvis Tabron

Published By **Jordan Levy**

Elvis Tabron

All Rights Reserved

*Hiit: Fastest Way to Burn Fat and Lose Weight
(Effective High Intensity Interval Training
Workouts, Exercises, and Routines- Hiit Workouts)*

ISBN   978-1-998769-07-0

No part of this guidebook shall be reproduced in any form without permission in writing from the publisher except in the case of brief quotations embodied in critical articles or reviews.

Legal & Disclaimer

The information contained in this ebook is not designed to replace or take the place of any form of medicine or professional medical advice. The information in this ebook has been provided for educational & entertainment purposes only.

The information contained in this book has been compiled from sources deemed reliable, and it is accurate to the best of the Author's knowledge; however, the Author cannot guarantee its accuracy and validity and cannot be held liable for any errors or omissions. Changes are periodically made to this book. You must consult your doctor or get professional medical advice before using any of the suggested remedies, techniques, or information in this book.

Upon using the information contained in this book, you agree to hold harmless the Author from and against any damages, costs, and expenses, including any legal fees potentially resulting from the application of any of the information provided by this guide. This disclaimer applies to any damages or injury caused by the use and application, whether directly or indirectly, of any advice or information presented, whether for breach of contract, tort, negligence, personal injury, criminal intent, or under any other cause of action.

You agree to accept all risks of using the information presented inside this book. You need to consult a professional medical practitioner in order to ensure you are both able and healthy enough to participate in this program.

TABLE OF CONTENTS

Chapter 1: Introduction To The Concept Of

Hiit

If you've been keeping track on the latest trends in fitness and trends, you're aware that HIIT continues to be a regular inclusion on these lists nearly every year. This is a testament to how beneficial it is for people looking to reach your fitness objectives without having to spend a lot of time in the gym.

While these workouts don't require a lot of time to complete but they could bring long-lasting improvements to your fitness and general health. Research has shown that HIIT will help you attain the same outcomes as exercise routines that are long and moderate in intensity accomplish.

What is the Science Behind HIIT

What happens when you're exercising at a level that your body cannot maintain for an extended period in time. Your muscle begin burning and it feels like you're running out breath. When you work out, your muscles begin to become awash in lactate and all the oxygen in your body becomes depleted.

The HIIT program makes your body work even harder to replenish the levels of oxygen in your blood. According to studies that your body works to replenish your store of oxygen up to up to 16 hours following having been off of exercise. Furthermore the HIIT training can increase your VO2 max , which is the body's ability to make use of oxygen as a source of energy. This improves endurance, and allows you to sustain long-term intense workouts longer than you believe you're capable of.

It's crucial to know that HIIT can improve both anaerobic and aerobic endurance, whereas moderate cardio workouts focus on your aerobic endurance.

A number of studies have also proven that HIIT workouts can help you burn off more calories throughout and after exercising, which allows you to lose weight quicker than if you were to do other types of exercises. Intensity of workouts will also cause a significant increase of catecholamines in your body. These are hormones that are activated whenever you're in a stressful situation. They're designed to in the mobilization of fat stores so that the body can use them to create energy.

Positive Benefits of the HIIT

The HIIT method is basically a short period of intense training which are then broken down by recovery and rest periods. For those who are just beginning it is important to know that you need to repetition exercises for about 20-30 minutes. This isn't only beneficial for those who don't have enough time to workout It's also an excellent method of cardio exercise.

Let's examine some of the benefits of HIIT will be available once you start this new exercise routine:

1. It can help improve your Blood Circulation

Training exercises that are based on intervals like HIIT could improve blood flow and dilation of blood vessels. According to studies, individuals suffering from the type 2 form of diabetes that engaged in HIIT saw significant improvements in their blood flow after an hour or two of exercising. The study also revealed that people who exercised had higher levels of glucose than those who didn't exercise as well as those who perform are doing steady-state or moderate intensity exercises.

2. It'll allow you to burn more fat

As we've seen that you're able to lose more calories in an HIIT workout than a steady-state exercise. It's equally important to keep in mind that this type of vigorous exercise can allow you to burn more fat over the following 24 hours as you would following running at a steady pace.

3. It can help you strengthen your cardiovascular Exercise

Because you'll be increasing your heart rate as well as the consumption of oxygen. These exercises will improve your cardiovascular and heart activity , and will also increase the amount of oxygen you consume and more specifically, your body's VO2 max. This is the amount of oxygen you'll need per kg of body weight. This can affect your stamina overall as well as your body's capacity to work out continuously.

Once you've become accustomed to the concept of HIIT and you'll see that you require less time for recovery in order to maintain your body in motion while burning off calories.

4. It can help in weight loss without building muscle

There's a downside to losing weight: you'll lose muscle mass and fat. While moderate intensity exercise promotes muscle loss exercising HIIT, weight training will enable for you to maintain your muscles in good shape, while also making it certain the pounds loss is due to the fat you store in your body.

5. It will help ease the aches and difficulties of Parkinson's Disease

University of Alabama published a study that suggests HIIT can improve functioning of the body, lifestyle and overall mental well-being of people suffering from Parkinson's. This could prove to be one of the most significant benefits of intense training when it's further studied as Parkinson's is a disorder that focuses on those motor abilities of the body.

In this study the researchers did not just observe improvements in balance and muscle control as well as their overall sense of wellbeing. The results were then compared to those who didn't engage in intense training.

6. It can increase your metabolism

HIIT can also boost the production of the human growth hormone by about 450 % within during the initial 24-hour period following exercising. The hormone is responsible for a higher calorific burn, and also aids in slowing the process of aging in your body. If you're concerned about your body aging too fast, try your HIIT routine now to reap the numerous benefits of interval training.

The HIIT Essentials to Recall

Once you've learned about the amazing advantages of HIIT when done correctly Let's look at the most important things you should consider prior to beginning to engage in HIIT. In this article we'll go over the amount of time you must perform the exercise, how intense this exercise should be in order to achieve the results you've hoped for, as well as the importance of rest and recovery time.

If you're just starting out and are not sure what to expect, HIIT can be quite efficient for you using your body weight. But, once you're to grips with it, you might need introduce certain equipment into your workout routine to ensure that you keep getting results.

You'll be shocked to know that HIIT is extremely versatile. It can be achieved using various techniques. It is possible to try biking and running on a treadmill. you could even incorporate ellipticals or bicycles in your exercise routine.

No matter which method, device or exercise you've chosen regardless of the method, machine, or activity you've chosen, be aware that you must perform it quickly and hard, and stop only whenever you feel that you're not able to continue or make your body go any further.

One popular choice that a lot of people opt for are treadmills. It's recommended that you choose the curved version of the treadmill because it can help you engage into a full-body exercise. You could also think about using stationary bikes since they can help increase the rate of your heart. A bike for arms is a great option for HIIT training that demands the most effort, which is why wrestlers have worked with for years to increase their endurance.

In order for your workout to be efficient, you'll need determine your personal intensity level. It's no surprise that the intensity of a beginner will differ from someone who's been exercising with this method for a long time. The sets are less in duration, between 20 and 90 seconds, however they will require you to use the full force of your body. If you've noticed that you are able to perform a set for more than half an hour, you're likely not exercising at the appropriate intensities.

While some might find it strange it is true that recovery and rest periods are vital in any exercise session that involves HIIT. If you do not take breaks to rest and recovery, you won't get the benefits of this exercise. The importance of rest periods is that your body must recover before you are able to contemplate doing another exercise.

It is important to note that the time of rest doesn't have to be complete rest. It is possible to have an active recovery time and take advantage of that time by doing the plank or walking in the same spot. Many fitness experts adhere to a 1:1 ratio, which means that for each minute of HIIT, it is recommended to be able to recover for two minutes.

Chapter 2: Improving Endurance With Hiit

If you're seeking to improve your endurance, contrary to popular opinion there is no need to spend hours a day working out and performing intense exercises. It is a excellent method to increase endurance since it targets key muscles that help build endurance.

Cardiovascular performance is the most important aspect of endurance. It is the way that your heart functions and how your circulatory system performs in response to the heart's pumps. The heart's functions can be assessed by using three factors:

1. Heart Rate

The heart rate refers to the number of your heart beating each minute. Your body is moving toward endurance quicker the more your heart beats each minute, and the more blood is circulated to the various organs in your body.

2. Stroke Volume

The term "stroke volume" refers to the quantity of blood circulated each when you beat your heart. Because endurance and your stroke volume are directly linked and a higher stroke volume is good for you.

3. Contractility

Contractility is the force your heart utilizes to pump blood into your body. If you experience greater contractility, that means that there is more blood flowing to your muscles. The blood is a source of oxygen and nutrients which your muscles of the skeleton require for durability and repair.

Why you should build Endurance

Endurance encompasses more than just an indicator of how well your heart is working to pump blood into your body. It is also a reference to the quantity of oxygen you are able to deliver into your muscle. Because our body and mind are quite connected when we work hard in physical exertion, our brains are stronger too.

Physical endurance can improve your brain's efficiency and have positive impact across all areas of your life and your physical well-being. Things like swimming, cycling or running demand endurance, so you'll continue to push yourself without getting tired. The term HIIT, which is also used to describe short bursts of intense training will help you build up your endurance, especially if you do it in conjunction with other types of training that are more traditional.

Utilizing HIIT to improve endurance

HIIT aids in building endurance by focusing your attention on all the aspects we've discussed in the previous paragraphs. It boosts the stroke volume to ensure that a sufficient quantity of blood is flowing to your muscles. Additionally it can have an effect on your contractility as well as the intensity of your heart's work to circulate blood.

It's also an excellent alternative to aerobic exercise in increasing the density of your mitochondria. If there are more mitochondria in your body that are more energetic, it provides and gives your muscles greater endurance, to work at a higher levels for longer, and also require less rest and recovery time.

HIIT aids in increasing the amount of enzymes found within mitochondria. As we've already established that energy is generated by various cycles within mitochondria. Different enzymes interact with the substrate to create products through all the steps involved in these cycles. Each of these enzymes is involved in their own distinct functions which are essential for the energy production. Because HIIT increases the amount the enzymes involved, these enzymes increase the endurance of your skeletal muscles.

When you engage in the HIIT exercise, it alters the signalling pathway inside your body , from slow rapid. To breakdown the nutrients and get energy out of mitochondria, they get activated through a switch in your body , known as PGCa. When you do intense exercise the signalling pathway intended to activate the switch is significantly faster. This leads to increased enzyme activity as well as an increase in mitochondrial density.

How HIIT helps build endurance in Skeletal Muscles

If you're doing these intense exercise, the vasculature which is the term used to describe the number and dimensions of blood vessels within the area that's in the skeletal muscle is altered. When you exercise the blood vessels that are tiny within your muscles of the skeletal system become more visible.

They pump more blood to your heart, which can help in enhancing the strokes of your heart. When muscles contract, they pump blood back into the ventricle of your left. The more blood that is transferred to the heart and back, the more it is oxygenated. This leads to an increased quantity of nutrients flowing into the muscles.

Additionally the high intensity training also builds endurance by increasing the endurance of muscles fibers. If you didn't know that muscle fibers are made from strands of protein. Because blood circulation becomes improved during these workouts More proteins are created from amino acids found within your blood. This improves the muscles' flexibility.

Exercises in HIIT for Endurance

Naturally, HIIT exercises are intensive and an ideal exercise choice for people with hectic lives that want to keep fit. They're a mix of short exercises that will aid in achieving a metabolic increase and maximize calorie burning that usually lasts for up to 48 hours after doing your workout.

Are you an athletic person in search of for a workout that will help with performance improvement, think about a mix of bodyweight exercises, plyometrics as well as a few challenging toning movements. Before beginning your routine it is recommended to do at least 5-10 minutes of cardio to warm up to make sure the muscles you're working ready for the rigorous workouts you'll be doing in the coming weeks.

How often do you need to perform these Workouts?

Because these routines are known for their high impact, they're kind of exercises that should be performed infrequently. It is recommended to perform them at least twice each week, and reserve the time for days when your schedule is crammed with work and don't have enough time to spend an entire 60-90 minutes in the gym. It doesn't mean you should not do cardiovascular or other exercises during the rest of the week however, it does mean that you need to select a style that is less abrasive on joints, as well as your other system.

When you're taking breaks from your HIIT routine it is recommended to do long-term endurance exercise. It could involve a gentle walk, 30-60 hours of walking a swim sessions or an elliptical.

Effect of Qmax increase after HIIT

Qmax is the highest amount of blood that could be delivered to your body within a matter of one minute. Research suggests that HIIT is not a significant impact on Qmax, while low-intensity exercises like aerobic exercises are proven to be efficient in improving Qmax.

This proves that HIIT uses cardiovascular pathways to aid in building endurance. It doesn't just boost the amount of mitochondria that are present within your cells, but enhances the function of the enzymes found within the mitochondria. No matter what how much you want to improve your fitness, your age, and your personal preferences for various kinds of exercises It is important to remember that moderation is essential. It is possible to incorporate HIIT as well as other types exercises into your workout routine to achieve the results you desire. It's important to keep in mind that the more varied your training routine is more varied, the easier it is for you to keep it up to date and not get exhausted or bored.

Chapter 3: Customizing Hiit And Making

Mistakes To Avoid

The benefit of HIIT is that it offers various combinations of exercises that you can choose from and they're completely customizable to the changing requirements and objectives. If you do HIIT often and select the appropriate type of exercise for you it will allow you to improve your fitness faster than any other exercise that are available.

A properly-designed HIIT program can increase your muscle mass and reap the benefits of cardiovascular exercise. It also helps to reduce the catabolic effects triggered by exercise routines that are more time-consuming. After you've improved your HIIT training it will allow you to lose weight, burn calories and achieve the body structure you've always wanted.

Who wouldn't be interested in the thought exercising and completing your routine in under 30 minutes? Although it may sound appealing, it's important to remember that HIIT is about pushing your body to its maximum which means it burns calories long after you've finished working out.

In order to ensure that your HIIT regimen is more efficient than ever before, it is essential to have some strategies in your mind. It's easy to get carried away when you're not as vigilant as you ought to be. Don't take the time to rest lightly, as they assist you in recovering from every workout and keep your body in shape.

If you're planning your workout schedule, it's important to figure out what you'd like to gain from it. According to the experts there are three primary physiological reactions that are triggered during high intensity interval training:

* Aerobic (enhancing your VO2 max)

* Anaerobic (high lactate levels)

* Neuromuscular (muscle recruitment patterns and soreness)

Before you decide on the best workout for you it is important to decide what of these aspects you're trying to activate. It's crucial to remember that this isn't a one-size-fits-all option, and you may select workouts that focus on two or all three these aspects.

You must be cautious because when you're a soccer player and you're undertaking mid-season conditioning don't choose exercises that cause your neuromuscular fatigue, as it could significantly hinder the performance of your team, therefore it's crucial to limit your workouts to shorter durations and make the most of recovery and rest periods.

Interval exercises can be divided into five types that are listed below:

• Short periods (these are expected to last between 10 seconds to one minute, with a the recovery time of less than a minute)

* Long periods (these should last between 2 and 5 minutes, with an interval of recovery of between 1 and 3 minutes)

* Sprints that are short (also called repeated sprints, which should last from 3 to 10 seconds and the recovery time of no more than 45 minutes)

*Long sprints (also called spring interval training, which is recommended to last between 20 seconds and one minute, with a resting period of between 1 and 4 minutes)

* Game-based exercise (this is usually a part of team sports that involve small-sided games, with intervals of rest in between)

As you might notice, each one of the exercises mentioned above have distinctive features which can be adapted in accordance with your objectives. Long sprints are primarily targeted at the neuromuscular and anaerobic systems, whereas longer intervals generate an anaerobic and aerobic stimulus within your body. They may even result in neuromuscular fatigue when you keep doing enough repetitions.

If this is your first time doing an HIIT exercise, you might want to modify it to match your fitness level, and having a 3 minute interval of rest for every four minutes of workout. After you've got used to the routine you'll start to see the results as you gain strength. Your recovery will be faster in time and you'll are able to decrease your time off between each workout. It's also recommended to utilize an electronic device to monitor your heart rate prior to and after your workout.

Common Errors to Avoid

It's not a fact that HIIT is a powerful workout however, if you're looking to achieve results, it's important to be doing it right. Because most people aren't accustomed to working their bodies to the extent they have to, even in an HIIT exercise that's just 7 to 10 minutes in length They often fall into mistakes that can sabotage their efforts, and stop their progress from being noticeable.

Let's examine some of the common mistakes to avoid when performing HIIT workouts:

1. Doing longer-lasting workouts

It's important to keep in mind that a good HIIT session could last anywhere between four and twenty minutes, or longer than thirty minutes if you're feeling like pushing it to the limit. If you're able to effortlessly push yourself past this amount of time, then it's not an accomplishment. The whole purpose of high intensity interval training is the fact that it doesn't need to do long sessions whenever you are able to challenge yourself to your highest limit within a short time of high-intensity interval training. This will make the duration of your workouts shorter when your body becomes exhausted enough to stop.

2. Not warming up properly

The HIIT training can be intense and demanding for people who aren't used to using the body's full potential when working out. Whatever your level and whether you're only starting out or practicing HIIT for several months it is important to prepare yourself before beginning your HIIT program.

It's a major mistake to head to the gym to begin by doing an HIIT exercise without warming-up beforehand since it could prevent you from experiencing the benefits you've been hoping for. If you don't warm-up beforehand, your body won't be able to maintain your body during the intense intervals and will cause you to get tired faster than you had hoped for.

3. Doing Not Pay Attention To "Recovery" Intervals

A common mistake made by people in HIIT is to shorten the rest or recovery time to make the exercise harder. This isn't the best option as the recovery time is as crucial, if perhaps more so, than the interval of high intensity. This is when your muscles take care of the debt known as oxygen which is the amount of oxygen that they didn't receive during the exercise that caused fatigue. Once they've gotten the oxygen back, they'll be in a position to work exactly the same amount of effort during the following session. If you don't give yourself enough time to recuperate then your muscles will be able to perform a portion of the next exercise.

4. Making Choices for complex movements

As per experts when you continue with your workouts the body can become exhausted enough to carry out complicated exercises. Beginning your first workout with the most complex movements may be the best idea initially but, over time, and with repeated exercises your body and mind may become over-exerted and increase the chance of injury, too.

It is recommended to opt for moves that are easier to perform to perform your HIIT workout. In this way, you won't have to give much focus on the direction your body part needs to go or what muscles you'll need to stretch out more.

5. It's not as hard as You'd Like

The issue to remember with HIIT practice is that you must challenge yourself so that, by the time you're finished with your high intensity workout you're exhausted and your heart is pounding in your chest. It shouldn't be possible to carry on after the timer is over. If this doesn't happen in your case, it shows that you're not performing a good enough job.

To allow your HIIT exercise to be successful you must be pushing yourself to the stage where your physical and mentally aren't able to push yourself further and you have to end the workout.

6. Making the wrong choice at the wrong time

Be cautious when choosing the timing to do your HIIT exercise. You shouldn't pick randomly one hour in the week to do the HIIT session. It is important to plan these sessions appropriately and ensure you're not doing them following a meal or before the time you go to bed.

It is best if you started training at the beginning of the day as you can. Consider eating a healthy but light breakfast just prior to starting your workout because this will enable you to focus on the fat reserves you have. It can also prepare your body for burning the calories you'll consume during the course of your day.

It's also important to keep in mind that HIIT will improve your productivity and concentration that's why it is important to exercise early before you go to work to boost your performance.

7. Doing HIIT every day

If you're eager to see the result of HIIT You could be doing it more often than you're supposed to. It's not good for the muscles of your body if you start performing HIIT each day. It's best to complete the HIIT routine at least twice or three times a week since it gives your body sufficient time to recover to prepare for the next session.

Many people choose this kind of exercise to long sessions of slow or moderate intensity training since it doesn't require the time to do it within their busy schedules.

Chapter 4: How To Make The Most Of Hiit

Through Corrective Exercises

If you're trying to make the most out of HIIT it is important to recognize the importance of combining it with appropriate and essential corrective exercises.

For the best results without risking of injury, you have to devote your days of recovery doing exercises that are corrective. We often begin the training session without taking joint issues or imbalances into consideration. We challenge ourselves to the limits of the limits of what our bodies are capable of, but we don't realize how it could negatively impact our overall health.

To put it into simple terms, we human beings live within the anterior chain of our bodies, which is the front of our bodies. All of our activities are in the direction of forward. This is why we have to do additional exercises that strengthen your posterior chain. It is necessary to increase the amount of reps performed on the posterior chain compared with the anterior chain. this is why the posterior chain is to overall fitness and health.

If, for instance, you push 10 times it is necessary to do 20 reps to target the posterior muscle. This could be any type of rowing exercises , like bands, ring rows, barbell rows and so on.

This is applicable to all types of exercises. If you're doing three chest exercises, you must pair it with three back exercises that twice the number of reps. You can do these reps with lighter weights so long as you're doing them. The reason you should double the reps is that they help to create new neural pathways within your muscles, making them stronger without the need to work out with heavy weight.

Understanding Pain

Similar to the majority of concepts about performance enhancement and training exercises for corrective purposes are usually more complicated than it has to be. It is essential to recognize your weaknesses and admit the cause before you identify the appropriate sort of corrective exercises and strategies to help your body you have to know the truth about general discomfort and ways to eliminate it efficiently.

The most straightforward method to achieve wellness is based on the idea that being healthy will aid in the elimination of discomfort. This is a proven fact. There's nobody in the world who's not benefiting from being stronger.

This is an amazingly simple and efficient method that everyone need to know about:

It's based on a basic Kinesiology-based approach that was lost in the mix of many other theories that have been developed over time. It's also known as push/pull also known as antagonistic balance.

Bodybuilders and athletes from all across the globe use this method of training because of the benefits to strength they can achieve through this simple idea. In simple terms that when you push, you must pull the opposite way to maintain stability. This is a method that bodybuilders rely on for muscle balance.

Louie Simmons of Westside Barbell is a coach who lives by this ethos and lives it to the max. He is a powerlifting trainer who has trained some of the best powerlifters around the globe using their Conjugate training method.

Instead of focusing on muscular balance for aesthetics the training of his is focused around strength and balance however, the two are found to be extremely alike. The way he trains concentrates more on building longevity rather than simply aesthetics.

Louie has often stressed that you must have a healthy posterior chain if you want to alleviate generalized pain. It's been observed that the majority of people are dominant in the front of their physique (anterior chain) and weaker posterior chains. Because we spend around 90percent of our time on the anterior side of the body all of our activities is focused on the forward. Even the most famous athletes spend the majority of their time working upon the anterior chain.

Here's a list of the things we do to utilize the anterior chain, or cut on the anterior chain, resulting in muscle imbalances. This involves endurance and strength training.

* Sitting

* Reading

* Work on your computer

* Texting while on your phone

* Consuming food

* Driving

* Running

* Biking

* Swimming

* Squatting

* Boxing

* Bowling

* Bench Press

* Yoga

* Brazilian Jiu-Jitsu

* Muay Thai

The list continues. This is just a sample of the many activities we engage in which constantly stress both our muscle and fascial systems to compensate for anteriorly.

Anterior chain dominance is determined to be the most significant cause of all pain. We spend a lot of time at a desk, reading, texting and driving and do nothing to correct it, and this is what causes issues, such as shoulder pain, knee pain, back pain. Many of us work or have life styles that require us remain in the anterior chain dominating position.

Patients who suffer from lower back pain and tightness generally have tightened tissues around their necks, chests and between the costals (around your ribs) and anterior delts and subscapularis. The body is conditioned to be straight, so much that our upper muscles begin getting tighter because they are trying to pull our shoulders to a straighter posture. This is often referred to as the 'tug of war result. It is

Many people are able to correct problems with pre- or post-workout foam rolling. It can be done through dynamic stretching and light bar work. It is important to ensure that your muscles are operating in a synergistic manner so that you can sustain your body throughout the workout and increase your performance. Corrective exercises can dramatically alter the way you perform and help you adapt to a challenging exercise schedule. If you're experiencing a glitch in your enthusiasm it will be difficult to execute your movements in a straight manner this is the reason why corrective exercise is essential.

Chapter 5: Balance Hiit Using Supplements

And Diet

Whatever workout regimen you're following, it's important to incorporate it into a healthy nutrition and supplements in order in order to reap maximum benefit.

Let's examine the supplements you need to think about incorporating into your diet in order to begin the healing process and gain the extra energy boost to be ready for intense workouts.

Greens Supplement

Greens Supplement will help you build strength and increase energy levels and is a crucial element for intense workouts. In the course of intense training the body starts to build up acid, which eventually slows down your performance and cause you feel tired. Due to the lactic acid that is produced by the body, pH levels start to fall which causes the mechanism that works within your muscles to cease functioning. That's where the Greens supplement can help. It will give you the power you require to continue when you've finished the session.

Caffeine

It's no secret that coffee aids in making your body better-aware, and that's the reason coffee is among people's most-loved morning beverage. It also makes you stay active and focused during your workout and improves your performance. However, this doesn't mean you have to take the caffeine in large quantities since it could be detrimental to your body. It's best to know your tolerance before you decide your daily consumption according to your tolerance.

It is recommended to consume about 300 grams of caffeine prior to starting in a rigorous workout to keep you energized.

Citrulline

Citrulline is another essential supplement that aids in the creation of nitric Oxide in your body. It also plays a vital function in controlling blood flow to your muscles as well as other organs. Since blood is comprised of oxygen and nutrients that are vital for general health and fitness The more blood flows into your muscle tissues, the better the muscles can draw energy from these nutrients.

It is important to note that in the presence of plenty of oxygen levels, muscles will be aerobically regenerated and produce a lower amount of lactic acid. This can result in increased energy and decreased fatigue.

Creatine Monohydrate

Creatine is an ingredient that's been extensively studied and utilized in a variety of sports supplements since its advantages were first identified. It has been discovered that creatine not only improves your athletic performance and improves your performance, but it also aids in increasing the amount of lean muscle mass that is present in your body.

It acts as a pH buffer which helps to regulate your pH throughout the day and ensures that your muscles are at the correct pH to perform at their best.

It's ideal for HIIT exercises because it permits your body to heal faster. Because it is essential to have breaks and recovery time in

HIIT training and when your body is able to recover at a higher rate it will allow you to perform more efficiently and achieve the best outcomes.

Combining these supplements with intense workouts can assist you in getting greater results sooner than you imagine. Make sure that you're taking the right quantities to achieve better results, higher levels of energy and shorter recovery times.

To benefit from your workout routine You must also adhere to a healthy diet that is compatible with your high-intensity training sessions. If you're doing the HITT exercise, you must consume a diet that is rich in protein and ensure that your carb intake is adequate. This will allow you to continue to push through tough workouts without giving in to fatigue.

It is also important to drink enough fluids to ensure you are productive. It is important to plan your meals before your workout carefully, to ensure that your body gets enough energy and time to recuperate between sessions. Be sure to include healthy fats in your post workout meals to reduce inflammation that could result from intense workouts.

Also, after you've finished exercising hard it's crucial to provide your body something that will replenish the energy that it's lost. Because your body has depleted glycogen reserves and your muscles are breaking down and you'll need to eat proteins for repair.

A good strategy is to incorporate the philosophies that is discussed in the eBook The Keto Diet Simplified in your daily diet along with your exercise to get the most outcomes faster. It is a high-protein and low carb diet which focuses on eating foods that contain sufficient amounts of protein, nutritious fats, and extremely few carbs. The purpose of this diet is to obtain more calories from fats instead of carbohydrates.

It does this by depleting your body of sugar reserves, and then breaking down fats and making it a fuel energy source. This causes the creation of ketones, a type of chemical that your body utilizes to fuel itself rather than glucose. There are many advantages when you try the keto diet, including improvements to your cardiovascular health, decreasing the chance of developing certain cancers and weight loss just to mention some.

In addition to eating in addition to food, you must fill in the water that your body has lost in the course of your exercise, so you must drink water throughout the day.

Whatever your ultimate goal in fitness is weight loss, or improved performance in sports, HIIT is the most effective solution. So long as you're doing the exercises properly and avoiding the mistakes that most individuals make and taking the necessary precautions and you keep seeing the results you've been searching for.

Rememberthat the time between rest and recovery between sessions are equally important and a balanced diet and taking supplements are vital if you are hoping to watch your body change into the body of your desires.

Chapter 6: How Hiit Works

The term HIIT is also referred to as high-intensity discontinuous workout also referred to as rapid making. This method of preparing can be applied to all kinds of fitness including swimming, cycling to home circuits. its merit is that it's easy and delivers amazing results in a short amount of time and efficiently, thereby reducing time. Because intensity is essential and essential, the most important aspect we need to examine is a framework that you can follow to control and monitor your levels of intensity, also that is known as the rate of Perceived Exercise scale (or RPE scale).

It's based on a rating one-to-10 scale. A 1 rating would be how you feel when sitting, which is it is not a lot of pressure to any extent of your imagination! The other end of the scale is an overall level of 10 that feels like you are physically pushed to your extreme. This outline allows you to continuously check to ensure that you're exercising at the appropriate level. The majority of us will for the part be working from levels 4 to 7 in the book. We can even reach level 8 in only two or three workouts. Each exercise will be based on the RPE level that you should work on in.

TWO WORKOUT AMPLIES:

Workout 1 45-Minute Power Walk

The workout is basically walking at a fast pace, which is, on the intensity level it would be at the level of four (moderate intensities). This speed is maintained throughout the entire 45 minutes. It is an intense workout that has health and fitness advantages.

Workout 2: 15 minutes Power Walk HIIT

This exercise would consist of two minutes of walking at a high intensity, that on the graph of intensity will be 4.5 and then 1 minute of walking as fast as you can and pushing the intensity to levels 6. 7.5. The intensity will feel extremely tough. Repeat this equation in a total of five times and the benefits are immense. In those brief 1-minute intervals, you'll be pushing yourself to your highest level levels, and that's how your body becomes stronger and more stable and produces amazing outcomes. Another benefit of this exercise is that you create the EPOC impact, but workout 1 isn't. In the end, out of both exercises, the one that will cause more weight loss and will have a more effect is workout 2.

Eliminate More Fat in a Shorter Time

In the event that you're required to consume fat to boost your health and overall health, then intervals ought to always be an element of your routine. In addition to being a clever method of completing an exhilarating workout, intervals work for changing your physique. Combining real-life intense effects with short recovery sections allows you to keep your training intensity at a high level while maintaining a remarkable structures. The appeal of high-intensity interval training is in its capacity to keep you burning calories even after you have left the area of focus. In essence, your body doesn't receive enough oxygen during periods of intense work. As a result you'll be accumulating some "obligation" for oxygen which must be paid back in the during your current workout to return to your normal. In the end, your digestion gets kicked in a long duration after your exercise. Health experts refer to this miracle as excessive post-practice oxygen consumption, also known as EPOC. The most exciting thing is that it is possible to integrate these amazingly productive active workouts into any busy life, and this book offers a wealth of workouts to look into. If you have events in which you're involved could even squeeze in the 5-minute HIIT exercise in a matter of minutes. No matter how busy your schedule is, you'll almost always have time.

TO RESULT IN WEIGHT LOSS

If losing weight is your aim it is important to be conscious of the calories you consume. The HIIT program is a fantastic fat-burning exercise, however, ultimately, losing weight boils down to a simple equation that is calories in against calories out. The quality of these calories is equally important. Although diets are an individual choice I suggest following a few rules if you're looking to shed weight.

Three meals are recommended a day.

Consume two to three small snacks between meals, including smoothies with protein, fresh veggies, or almonds. These snacks should contain between 100 and 200 calories.

* Ensure your meals and snacks have an excellent source and supply of protein lean. It is the primary ingredient that makes up muscle. Remove alcohol.

Eliminate sodas as well as coffee beverages that contain sugar and other high-calorie sweet drinks.

Avoid eating foods that contain refined white sugar or flour. The following guidelines will allow you to stay clear of the heavily refined, simple carbohydrates that your body quickly converts into fat.

Limit your carbs to simple, unprocessed carbs like sweet potatoes.

Drink plenty of fluids. It helps flush the body of toxins and will keep you satisfied.

How YOUR BODY Moves

The most important aspect of any workout program is to utilize the same amount of moving planes as you can in order to achieve astonishing outcomes. There are numerous exercises that are centered around a specific area of movement. The consequence is that they over-burden the muscle groups that focus, which can cause injuries, and inversely affecting posture. Additionally If training and chiseling your body is something you require then utilizing 3 planes of motion is essential because it cuts and ensures your safety from every edge.

The three planes are:

*Sagittal (which is forward and reverse motion) It is the most frequently used plane.

*Transverse (which is an bending or rotational movement).

*Lateral, also referred to being the frontal (which refers to the sideways move).

The sagittal plane is by far the most widely-known movement plane that we do not just training, but also every day life. It is basically pushing the body forward or reverse.

The exercises are executed in the sagittal axis: paddling, strolling, running and cycling, lunges, push-ups, squats and squats. In the event that you tried an exercise that consisted of running, and then at some time, squats or push-ups will be the only thing you'll ever work your muscles through the sides and the back of your body, and moving through all of your muscles on your sides.

Frontal movements are taking the movement towards the side, and it is utilized often in racket sports where you move towards the side or hit the racket by moving your arms towards the side. It is also used utilized in various exercises, such as skating lunges, or the well-known star bounce. (Utilized in HIIT exercises This is an amazing sidelong move that is, in reality that this diamond travels across all of the facets.)

In the end, at last , transverse is an axis of rotation, and the most common examples of this would be boxing, golf or certain types of swimming. Additionally, a remarkable example of this workout is an Ab Shaper, which is a part of the 7-minute HIIT Workout since it targets your muscles on your sides, the inner and external obliques which help to draw the midriff.

When you exercise it's beneficial to make sure that you're using at all time two movements.

DURATION Vs. INTENSITY

Additionally, INTENSITY comes out at the top, which makes fitness classes with HIIT the top priority.

Like everything else in life the more you put in, the more successful your results. A 7-minute HIIT exercise at home in contrast to a 30-minute delicate bike ride at the fitness center will give you many more benefits, because the short bursts of high intensity are the ones that have the greatest impact on the surrounding.

* Increase the capacity of your body to metabolize fat

• Increase your cardio-vascular health

Reduce the feeling of anxiety.

* Reduce time

* You are able to continue the exercise in your daily life

* Tone all over the place

* Feel astounding

* The maturing process is slowed down.

* Improve your general health

* Finally, you will be energized and radiate vitality constantly

FIT tests and results

RESULT INSPIRED YOU TO WORK

Perhaps the most powerful motivational factor is seeing results, and by using the help of this HIIT publication, you could expect to see them quickly and in your body shape and how fit you are. To achieve this, I recommend that you take the exercises that come with it and keep a record of repetitions or times. It is possible to choose just one of them, or you may have to try different combinations. Try these tests again every 3 weeks, and I'll tell that on the possibility that you've been working out, you'll get amazing results.

The 1-Mile Test A ONE-MILE TEST: RUN OR WALK

In this test, you could either walk or run but you must follow the course for one mile and complete the separation within as little time as you are able. If you're no longer a youngster to exercise then, you can continue walking and take your time. If you're a runner you should run at your fastest speed. Note Date, Time and the way you felt (e.g. exhausted, depleted, or thinking that it was straightforward).

The upper body test THE UPPER-BODY TEST: PULSH-UPS

For middle to advanced exercisers and amateurs do the exercise using your knees. For the most advanced exercisers complete the full body workout. Push-ups are an excellent way to assess your upper body strength and endurance. Do as many of push-ups you can in a good form and take notes of the number of them you are able to do. You'll be surprised to observe the number increase in approximately three weeks.

The lower body test: WALKING LUNGES

Lower body muscles will quickly increase stamina and endurance and an excellent way to determine this is performing the walking lunge test. You should first determine the number of lunges that you can perform, you are still performing them using a an excellent technique. Each time you complete exercises, you'll enhance and increase your lower-body fitness. You'll be thrilled with the improvement that you notice every time you take the test.

THE LIST OF YOUR HIIT KIT HIIT

The best part about HIIT can be that it requires require just your body and an exceptional mental state to achieve an unimaginable exercise. However there are a handful of pieces of equipment that can improve your comfort when you're working out your execution.

FOOTWEAR

When you exercise It is essential to be aware of the location of your feet as you walk. Poorly-planned positioning can lead to an unsecure base for your body and cause injury. To ensure that you are more conscious of your foot's position and posture, wear a minimalist style shoe while exercising.

Two models specifically designed for HIIT include the Nike Free 1.0 Cross Bionic and INOV-8's F-Lite range of footwear. If you're not used to minimalist shoes it is recommended to change between your previous sneakers and the minimalist ones for a period of around 14 days, which allows your body to adjust to the reduction in padding and back.

YOGA MAT

It's possible to make use of an exercise mat to do floor exercises. It's a good way to keep your feet on the ground and could be more suitable for exercises performed in the back.

TIME OR WATCH

A timer or watch is essential for keeping track of the rest and work intervals in HIIT schedules. Use the device that's comfortable and easy to use, no matter whether it's a game-watch or a pulse screen or a mobile phone app which allows you to schedule intervals.

TOWEL

HIIT can get you sweat-soaked! Keep a towel nearby to remove sweat from your forehead and ensure that your work area is dry.

FOAM ROLLER

Foam rollers are an effective device that can provide myofascial release in the same way as static stretching or back rub. The use of a froth roller can prevent damage and speed recovery post-workout.

OPTIONAL EXTRAS

The HIIT program is linked to making use of many muscle groups in a manner that is prudent one in quick, unpredictable exercises. Utilizing segregation exercises like Bicep twists are restricted. In the case of certain exercise routines, it's okay to push yourself with the weight. You can also add some protection to exercises such as Russian twists, V-ups and sprinter sit-ups using an arm or portable weight or a drug ball.

Find a place in the home and use it to create your own exercise area. If you are able to, store everything on your checklist in this space and ready to go when you're prompted to perform one of my HIIT-based workouts. Additionally, at last, put on a dress. The most essential workout tools included in the kit list here are the coaches as well as the sports bra. When it comes to your workout equipment the most important aspect is that you are comfortable and at ease. If you're working out outside, ensure you're an area that is easily noticed.

Utilizing Tools and Toys

The use of fitness equipment that is portable for HIIT is an amazing approach to make the workout more challenging that is varied, as well as focus on different elements of fitness, like quality, perseverance and power. Equipment, such as medicine balls, stability balls suspension trainers, tubing smaller than regular trampolines, the skimming circle, ironweights and free weights are a great way to add an amount to your body weight exercise routines. This is the safe and effective usage of equipment and toys during HIIT exercises.

Why do we need tools and Toys?

Sometimes referred to as toys or tools portable fitness equipment could provide a lot of strength, variety as well as a boost and focus specifically body parts for the HIIT exercises. Although it's a fundamental body mechanics that are without any equipment, focusing during all HIIT grouping is crucial equipment may also bring enjoyment and involvement. For instance, medicine balls may help to build endurance and strength in the chest region. Stability balls could provide a unique challenge to the push-up. Being free of the floor can provide an alternative chest and middle problem. Tubing can provide a different perspective to the competition preparing for a particular body component.

These tools are moderately light and portable. They are easy to store and use, and can be a big help to the process of focusing and challenge while you are preparing.

If you don't have the tools or toys, you can get HIIT training using bodyweight exercises, where equipment is not needed.

Tools and Toy Safety

If you are using equipment during HIIT exercises security and safety should be your primary concern. The way you utilize equipment is an important consideration. The tools and toys you use should enhance the experience, not distract from the experience. If they're not making the exercise more exciting or offering a unique of a kind challenge they could not be helpful. Because HIIT conventions are often physically demanding with high-impact and horizontal movements and advancements ahead equipment in the vicinity could become an obstruction or a risk. If you are using portable equipment, you should move it away from the path of your body's movement to avoid walking on it or falling over it.

The following is a summary of the main points for the safe play with toys and tools:

Please read the instructions for proper usage of and weight limits for equipment and toys, like the stability balls and suspension trainers.

• Be aware of your goals, abilities and capabilities, as well as any previous injuries or obstacles.

Choose weights or loads that you are able to control regularly.

* To avoid sliding and dropping your equipment clean off equipment that has become wet from sweat.

• Keep all equipment away from the paths of moving vehicles when it is not in use.

Toy and Tool Options Toy Options

Of the numerous tools and equipment you can utilize in HIIT exercises, it can be difficult to determine what is the best option for you, based on your fitness goals and preferences, as well in the context of what you can access. In the following paragraphs, we will discuss many different tools and toys that can be utilized in HIIT exercises, such as size and weight guidelines and what they're most suitable for.

Stability Balls

Stability balls provide assistance and challenges during upper and lower body exercises. They also offer resistance and stability exercises for fundamental exercises. Balls that are burst-safe and have a diameter of between 55 and 65cm (22 or 26 inches.) are suggested.

Tubing for Resistance Tubing

Tubing for resistance provides continuous challenge and strength in multiple planes and is suitable for lower or upper body exercises. In addition, fundamental stability training often is a requirement when using tubing for resistance. Tubing use in various methods can reflect real-world changes, thus making it easier to practice the aspects of training.

Medicine Balls

Medicine balls are utilized to help with upper-body pulling and pushing development, as well as endurance or strength-based core exercises as well as rotational development. They also help to provide weight to the lower part of the body during squats or spins, or when throwing. Balls that are light weight for medicine are great to use. Stick with 2four, 6- as well as 8-pound ball (somewhere between 1 and 4 kilograms).

Tubing is available in long lengths with handles or in a figure eight shape. The resistance changes as its length exactly as much as the thickness. Shading is a typical method of demonstrating the degree of resistance.

Suspension Trainer

A suspension trainer is an outstanding method of training the upper, lower body, as well as the core. Once it is moored, the suspension trainer incorporates cardio, flexibility, strength and continuous in a HIIT workout. Suspension training is based on gravity as well as the positioning of the body with respect to the staying point. There are several models for suspension-training equipment are offered but TRX suspension trainers have become most popular and are typically used for training with body weight. Suspension trainers are more intense expectation to learn and adapt, and require more supervision than other tools and toys, but they are able to be received with ease and quickly mastered.

A bit smaller than normal Trampolines

Individual wellness trampolines or trampolines that are smaller than regular ones, are a fantastic alternative for training with high-power as they take away a significant portion of the ground reaction forces during high-sway bounces, and they also they take into consideration significant strength and challenge. There are many trampolines that can accommodate up to 350 pounds (159 kg) of body weight. They come in spring-stacked and string-joined models. An effective strategy is vital when using trampolines in HIIT exercises to achieve the right exercise performance to get over the anaerobic edge. For instance, it's crucial to know the best way to push down or load down when using the trampolines, instead of jumping up.

Gliding Disks

Gliding disks are small fabrics or plastic disks which slide across the floor. They can provide the force and intensity to almost every exercise that targets the upper, lower or the core, such as like blasts, bouncing jacks and push-ups. They are roughly similar to a plate and glide smoothly across the floor when they are properly positioned. Paper plates or towels could be used in place of gliding disks. Towels work well on wood surfaces and paper platesfor surface that is covered.

Kettlebells

Light kettlebells are a fantastic upgrade to strengthen the structure for endurance, power, and continuance control of movement; as well as traversing multidimensional planes. Kettlebells are amazing for increasing grip strength and regulating the energy that is required, which calls for massive core responsibility and full body involvement. Since kettlebells can be swung, they are not the only thing to consider. The body responds differently when an iron weight is used more than it does to a weight that is free with regards to controlling joints and connecting to the core muscles.

Due to the rapid-paced exercise of HIIT kettlebells with a light weight are recommended 4, 6, 8 10, 12 as well as 15 pounds (somewhere between 2 to 6 kilograms).

Free weights

Free weights can increase strength, endurance, stamina and definition in the working muscles. They can be a significant burden for exercises within an HIIT routine. Hand weights can be a secure and powerful method to combine the strength training and cardio workout. Be sure to use weights that you are able to control. 8 10 12 15- and 20-pound (somewhere between 4 to 9 kilograms) weights are ideal for this type of exercise.

Toys, gadgets and other small equipment are useful in HIIT workouts as they give the possibility of a variety and additional challenging. They're also useful due to the fact that dynamic training examples can be a significant boost to HIIT training results and in general exercises are more engaging. Tools and toys also allow users to focus on particular areas of your body for increased endurance in addition to better muscle tone development, and increased endurance while doing the HIIT.

HIIT and other FORMS OF EXERCISE

CIRCUIT TRAINING VS HIIT

Although HIIT is able to utilize a part of equipment and activities that are indistinguishable like high-intensity training however, the main difference with aerobics is that it uses low in power and there are no recuperations that are timed. In high-intensity aerobics, you simply start with one exercise and then move on to the next without a recommended time of rest during the middle. High-intensity exercise, generally speaking involves activities that require opposition like hand weight presses and weighted squats that are incredible for building quality and healthy muscles. However however, the aim isn't to force yourself into the high-force zones of training.

In this regard high-intensity exercise doesn't offer the same benefits for cardio as HIIT and does not cause the EPOC impact that causes you to consume calories for a long time after the workout has ended. According to NHS guidelines, adults should do two sets of opposition-based exercises each week, focusing on slenderness and structure, as well as increasing the thickness of our bones. In this manner, quality exercise that is high intensity and based on strength is an excellent addition of your fitness routine However, it should not be confused with HIIT-training.

HiIT Vs LISS

In contrast to HIIT that we are aware of, HIIT is focused on short, sharp intervals and clock-based recovery. LESS or Low Intensity Steady State (LISS) exercise is on the other side of the spectrum when it comes to training. There are those who arrive at the fitness center and take a straight route to the closest curving coach and take an entire hour to stir up a sound "sparkle" while reading the most current issue of Hello magazine? Absolutely, that's LISS. However, while there is the possibility to consume calories while doing a LISS workout, the benefits end once the workout is completed. A long, low-power workout isn't going to send your digestive system into high gear, resulting in an the most significant impact after consumption. In the event that you're a endurance athlete with specific goals you're in the direction of, LISS may be a element of your fitness plan. If in any the event that you're an exercise enthusiast who wants to take their fitness to the next level and really alter your body's shape You'll definitely gain benefit in less time by doing an HIIT exercise.

Who is HIIT for?

The majority of people will have no issues with HiIT.

The Person Who Has Been Trained

For the more experienced, HIIT will allow you to enhance your abilities and at a faster rate. HIIT can allow users to evaluate their skills to the highest level. If you believe you're cardio-fit but haven't implemented any form of HIIT into your routine You'll become accustomed to HIIT quickly and have no trouble adapting. The sudden shock to your frame will force your body to make these improvements to your fitness in a rapid pace that you've never seen through CT. I'm putting my trust in and fully anticipating that you will become an advocate and supporter of HIIT.

The Individual who isn't trained

If you're not active or do not exercise regularly then it's always recommended to consult an expert prior to embarking on a fitness program to ensure that you're physically in good shape to participate. This applies to any new exercise routine that is not only HIIT. It is important to make sure you are aware of this because the primary purpose of the HIIT program is to achieve higher levels when compared with other types of training but for shorter time periods. Although the evidence suggests that you can perform HIIT in a moderate level in the beginning, the objective is to always get as intense as you can, which is 100% of your maximum heart rate. Ideally, you should also be aiming to maintain this level of intensity for as long that you are able to.

The growth of lactic acid within your muscles, as well as the use of CP stores is the primary aspect in determining to what degree you'll be able to sustain this intensity, and the degree of it will differ for every individual. It is possible to progress to this point but it has to be understood that it's where you're supposed to get there earlier, and the quicker the more beneficial. Therefore, if you're a novice it is best to start with the simplest end of the range. It is possible to do this by making your high-intensity workouts slightly less memorable and with a shorter time. You are able to choose the length of your recovery intervals, making sure that it's suitable with your particular body. With a couple of HIIT sessions You'll be able to increase the intensity, and be amazed by the speed at which your health increases.

If you're worried about achieving the level of exertion required It is likely that there will come a time in your life when you'll have to perform bursts of intense and high-intensity and speedy exercise. Consider the time you're rushing to catch an airplane or train carrying two heavy baggage packs. Maybe you've got an emergency in your family that you have to address and you're required to get at home as fast as you can. It's not a question of the amount of work required to make it home in these circumstances. What happens if someone takes your backpack and wallet, or your mobile phone? Wouldn't it be awesome if you were trained to be prepared for those times when you would need it?

Of course, you'll end up leaving plenty of gas in your tank as you start and will be slipping through the difficult and fast HIIT routine within a half-month. There is no one who would like to see you become an Olympic athlete in the near future. However, when things get easier for you, which they will it is best to be able to count on the intensity but not the length of the workout. This is not the case with CT in that the intensity is the key word to enchantment and not the duration. Quantity not quality!

The busy individual

For those who live hectic schedules, HIIT can help you achieve every benefit of a longer exercise routine in less duration. Because of the long durations of wellness advice and recommendations of health advice, many people are unaware that losing weight and improve the health of their body and heart require a significant amount of constant training, which takes an enormous amount of time. Studies show that the most one reason for resistance to workouts is the lack of time. When you're using HIIT you can never be blamed. If you're the kind of person who spends much of their time in work, residing in lodgings or in the middle of a vacation then you can be sure that using HIIT, you'll have no requirement for equipment and, in certain instances you don't need an enormous amount of space as well.

BEFORE YOU STARTE the HIIT

Wellness Assessment

Before you begin HIIT it is important to know your current health level. The basic wellness assessment will help you determine where to start and provide a framework for estimating your progress. The wellness appraisal is comprised of four basic exercises: push-ups, X-jacks Squats, sprinter sit-ups. Before starting, review the instruction of each workout. Then, add these signifies:

1. Perform each exercise for 30 seconds.

2. Pause for 30 seconds at the end of each exercise.

3. Make a note of your reps were able to complete for every exercise in the 30 second interval (for example twenty squats).

4. Add the total number of repetitions completed for each exercise to calculate your final score.

When your scores are:

* 1-80 - Begin with level 1 schedules.

* 81-104 - Begin by following The Level 2 schedules.

* 100+ - Begin with the level 3 schedules.

BODY FAT Percentage

HIIT has been proven experimentally to burn body fat as well as it creates slender muscle. Since muscle is more sensitive than fat, simply observing your weight may be a bad indicator of your progress when you are doing HIIT. Calculating the body fat percentage could be a better method of evaluating your the results. There are a variety of methods to estimate body fat, with some being more accurate than others. I recommend using tape measures and the military method that is the formula used in the U.S. Branch of Defense for estimating the body fat percent.

GET YOUR MEASUREMENTS

Make use of a tape measure to note the boundaries of your waist, neck, and hips. You can measure in centimeters or inches.

Neck.

Take a look at your neck's periphery. It should be an area just below the larynx (Adam's apple) and in the opposite direction to the long pivot of your neck. Then round it up to the nearest one half centimeter (half one inch).

Waist.

Take a look at your waist's normal outline by rubbing your skin in the area of the tightest point of your belly. It is usually approximately halfway between your navel, and at the bottom portion of your chest (bosom bones). Make sure that the tape is straight and in line with the ground. The measurement should be rounded up to the closest 1/2-inch (or one half-centimeter).

Hip.

Take a measurement of your hip's circumference and do not use the estimating tape to determine the largest piece of your glutes when you look at the back. Be sure that the tape is in line with the ground. Make sure you round up the measurement of your hip to the closest half centimeter or half inch. Also, you will need to measure your height in centimeters or inches.

Chapter 7: Hiit Versus Continuous Training

I came up with the ideal way to begin this book is to convince readers to highlight the huge gap in possible accomplishments in the case of comparing HIIT and CT by examining a variety of exercise routines. You'll discover that HIIT is superior to CT in all aspects. Let's now think about two techniques for preparing the following areas:

* Exercise and Fun

* Weight Loss

* Exercise Duration

* Increased Fat Burning

* Capacity Anaerobic

* Threshold

* Beta-Endorphin Levels

* Maximal Oxygen Uptake/VO2 Max

* Athletic Performance

Exercise and Fun

When most people start exercising they realize the fact that CT is the primary kind of high-impact exercise that it is possible to do, even though there are a myriad of options to do CT including treadmills cycling, paddling skiing, stair climbing, circular coaches and so on. In light of the usual fitness advice novice exercisers receive they imagine a long time working away in front of the clear line. For a lot of people, CT before long gets boring. Training at the same, or at the bare minimum, levels for more than 45 minutes is a little boring for the majority of the population. Numerous studies have shown that exercise fatigue is among the primary reasons that people give up. You're sure to feel this. What could be more boring than sitting on a stationary fitness bike (or the supplement equipment there) over 45 minutes trading at the same rate and with the same power for the whole time?

HiIT is definitely more exciting because you can always change the speed. The casual conversations with customers prove that instead of dreading the idea of an exercise session, they are anticipating the concept of the idea of a HIIT session and all it entails. There's something extremely relaxing about running at full speed for a couple of minutes before taking a slow walk, and then before accelerating to maximum speed for a second.

One issue that comes with CT can be that the thought of being just at ten minutes into your run and then having more than 30 minutes left and running at the same pace is motivating. However, with HIIT, knowing the fact that you've been running a remarkable speed for two seconds prior to taking a easy stroll for a few minutes, for example is a pleasant experience to the brain and could spur your energy levels in a way that isn't clear. The process of working at high levels is much easier when you notice that you're taking an opportunity to rest at the next corner. This could be confirmed by examining a research study conducted in Liverpool John Moores University in the year 2011. The goal was to consider how enjoyment is perceived by the groups that participate the same experience in HIIT and another group who participated in CT.

The main group of eight men completed 6 high-force intervals thirty seconds, at 90% maximum heart rate. These intervals were combined with three minute intervals of walking at a slow pace. The next group continued to run through 50 mins at a steady pace that was equal 70-80% of the maximum heart rate. Everyone surveyed their satisfaction using their Physical Activity Enjoyment Scale. The scale consists of 18 questions where participants assess their satisfaction using an scale from 1 to 7.

The higher the score - the greater the level of enjoyment. Evaluations of perceived enjoyment for the HIIT group were assessed as 88 while the CT group scored their enjoyment at 61. This was despite the evaluations of perceived effort that were barely higher in those in the CT group. But, for those reading this book and who regularly take seriously a fascination with HIIT as well as those who are about to learn that HIIT is more enjoyable simply because of the fact that HIIT can be more enjoyable than continuous preparing shouldn't cause any alarm.

Weight Loss

Research has shown that when it comes to the loss of weight, HIIT can be superior to CT. In the University of Western Ontario in the year 2011, 20 participants were randomly assigned to either a HIIT group or the CT group. Within the HIIT group, participants were expected to run on a treadmill for between 4 and 6 instances of full-scale dashes lasting 30 seconds. Each 30-second period of complete dashing was accompanied by intervals of recovery lasting up to 4 minutes. The CT group exercised on treadmills at a rate that was 65% of their maximum heart rate for an amount in the 30 to an hour. Instructional classes for both groups took place three times a week for six weeks. What were the results?

Following the study of 6 weeks subjects of the CT group shed a total of 5.8 percent in their body fat. This is a remarkable result. However should there not be something to say concerning this HIIT group? The subjects of the HIIT group lost a total of 12.4 percent from their body fat. Do not be afraid to read the study for yourself (all studies used within this publication are cited in the end of the book). The results prove that HIIT is an undisputed groundbreaker over CT in terms of weight loss or fat loss. at least, this is the case when you are interested in HIIT sessions three times per for a period of 6 weeks like in the study. However is it true that taking part in high-power activities result in a greater number of outcomes when they are performed regularly over a longer time frame?

Let's examine another study. In the year 1990, The American Journal of Clinical Nutrition examined data out of the Canada Fitness Survey. The survey included 1366 males and 1257 females aged between 20 and 49 were assessed for body fatness and weight distribution (waist measurement of hip to waist) as well as energy consumption as well as frequency, intensity, and duration of routine leisure-time activities. All data were gathered through the use of a comprehensive questionnaire and also through physical measurements made in an environment of clinical. To assess the impact of intensity and exercise on body fat percentage subjects of both sexes was divided into 4 groups taking into consideration that the metabolic equivalent to task (METS) importance of their leisure-time activities.

Group A - subjects who are not reporting activity of 5 METS or higher Group B - between 5 and 7 METS. Group C between 7 and 9 METS group D - those who report activities that are 9 METS or greater.

Before I present the results, let's take an look at some examples of METS value examples. When you sleep, you score a METS value of 0.9 and walking at 3 miles per hour (4.8 km/h) will give you a number of 3.3 METS. However, for reasons of HIIT, sprinting, or rope jumping will give an METS score of 10. Each activity has been assigned an METS score that grades the intensity of physical activity specific activity. If you're interested in the intensity of your work or your favorite pastimes are you can simply conduct an online search to find The Compendium of Physical Activities.

The study's results revealed that participants in group D was the most slimmest group, with the lowest waist-to-hip ratio, the smallest waist circumferences, and the smallest body fat percentages compared to all other groups, and for both genders. This was regardless of the fact that group D used an equal amount of energy for activities, as did group A, but less than the participants in groups B and. We'll clarify that the study found that the participants in the group D used the same amount of energy when they engaged in the same activities as group A (but lower than group of B and C) but their body composition was completely different. There are many other variables that are at play here, and we'll certainly discuss them in the near future.

Why is HIIT more effective for the loss of weight CT? There are two major reasons to explain this. It's been long-known in physiology that if you intensify the workout, you boost the speed of metabolic breakdown of carbohydrates and consequently reduce metabolic rate for fat. If you're looking to shed weight or, more specifically, you're looking to shed weight, then this is against your goals. But, when you increase the intensity of your exercise it also increases the caloric consumption rapidly.

If you burn more of fat calories through exercises with lower intensity The total amount of calories from fat is much lower because of the lesser total number of calories burned in the workout. In contrast, if you increase your intensity, you'll burn off an enlargement of fat calories, yet with more caloric expenditure. If you look at the logic behind this the less percentage for a larger number is much greater than a higher percentage of a lower percentage. There are numerous health professionals who aren't sure about this reasoning and their clients and patients don't benefit from high intensity exercise. It's logical to conclude that by performing lower-intensity exercise, people would be losing more carbohydrate to fat than doing more intense exercises and thus this strategy appears to be superior to lose weight. When you consider the amount of energy expended while exercising, this idea is plausible at a certain level.

However the fact is, as we begin to realize that this isn't true. Naturally, a variety of variables are involved such as the post-exercise process. The post-exercise processes are frequently ignored even by human services experts and many fitness coaches specifically in the context of cardio-training. Another instrument is excessive oxygen consumption after exercise (EPOC). If you don't have difficult to read the section titled Improved Fat burning capacity below since we'll discuss EPOC in great detail. Another thing to note Consider taking a second look at the research in the above study. There's something in that study that any sharply glanced at user is likely to have noticed. This leads us to the next sub-heading.

Exercise Duration

Have a look at the word exercising in each of the subject categories mentioned above. What are you able to see? While reading this study you'd believe there was mistake. For the study to be sensible, the two groups would have needed to be able to use comparable exercises, however this wasn't the case. In the study the CT group worked out for a typical 45 minutes per session.

Compare that with the HIIT group, which exercised for a typical duration that was 22.5 minutes for each session. It's true that the HIIT group was exercising for less time that those in the CT group. But, by the time they had completed of the study and participants took their body fat levels checked again and again, the HIIT group had seen a decrease of more than two times in weight. This was more than twice what they had lost. CT groups had shed 5.8 percent for the CT group and 12.4 percent for the HIIT group.

The research suggests that you can shed more than twice the amount of body fat by completing significant portions of your exercises using HIIT in comparison to CT. Practically speaking it means you can reduce your HIIT session considerably and reap benefits that are superior to any lengthy and boring CT session. Do you believe that you're beginning to realize the advantages of HIIT in the present? I invite you to look over the study yourself. What is the primary reason why the vast majority of people promise that they will not engage in any health-related activities?

It's not due to lack of motivation or money however, rather lack of time is the reason. Utilizing HIIT and HIIT, you will reap greater benefits than CT using only a tiny part of the time put into it. Since I have noticed different studies in this book, if it's not too hard to keep track of the terms for exercise that the 2 study teams because this will help to emphasize the point made above. We've set up the idea for you to know that your HIIT sessions don't have to take that long to achieve astonishing and perhaps even better benefits over CT. But, how much time in the week do you need to put into it? What amount of exercise sessions are it advisable to take part in order to reap these advantages? As you can see from the research above the past year, a 12.4 percent reduction in the amount of fat was achieved in just three separate sessions each week (for six weeks). I'm sure I don't have to reveal to you just the magnitude of this study.

In any event I'll refer you to a study which examined the effects of one episode in HIIT each week, on the mortality rate of cardiovascular disease with cardiovascular disease being the primary cause of deaths across the world. This study was awe-inspiring in that it analyzed 56,000 individuals across a long time. The results showed that to prevent cardiovascular disease the single weekly HIIT session significantly reduced the risk of dying in two individuals. It was interesting to note that extending either the duration of a single HIIT workout or the frequency of weekly HIIT workouts had none of the benefits that were added in counteracting the effects of death due to heart disease. The study suggests that, if weight reduction isn't your primary goal then all you require is one 22.5-moment session each week to achieve this. In general, one could now to cite lack of time as the motive for not exercising?

Better Fat Burning

It's been established that the more you exercise, the greater weight-loss capacity your body can create for itself. What I mean is that the longer you work out, the after some time, your body turns into a more efficient in consuming fat, regardless of the time you're on the town , taking part in your normal work or at any other event, even if you're in the sofa watching a film. Why is that? There are a number of internal mechanisms in the body that can provide the defense.

Increment in Mitochondria

One of these mechanisms is the increase in the amount of and size of mitochondria that are present in muscle cells. Mitochondria are often referred to as the cells that "control houses" because they are where glycogen is transformed into vitality and oxygen is created. If you exercise, over a period of time, the increase in mitochondria and the effectiveness increases the body's ability to eat fat. So , how does this expanded limit compare with HIIT or CT?

We need to look into another study. In the University of Guelph, Ontario in 2008, the study was planned to examine HIIT and its potential to increase the body's metabolic fat and starch limitations in people who have not been trained. The participants took part in 10 times of high force cycling separated by two-second recovery periods. The exercise sessions were conducted three days a week for six weeks. At the end this study resting muscular biopsy was performed and there were a number of changes of citrate synthase (26 percent) the mitochondrial chemical, and two distinct fat-carrier proteins (14 percent and 30 percent). It was found that when the rate of cycling was constant at 60% maximum potential for pulses it was evident that there was an increase in starch and fat ability to oxidize.

The most shocking thing about this study is that it did not examine the contrast between HIIT subjects with CT subjects, which would have been interesting to observe. In order to clarify the results, the test revealed that the increase in carbohydrate oxidation abilities was specific to CT exercises that were performed after HIIT sessions. It is evident that after of doing HIIT for a time and then returning to CT the body's body has proven to be becoming more efficient in eating fat. Another study conducted at a similar university in 2006, eight women took part in 10 sessions of high-force cycling with recovery times of two minutes. Participants participated in seven exercises over a 14-day duration. At the end of the study the fat oxidation capacity were up by 36%..

Unfortunately, it was not a CT group to compare results with. It's likely that they completed their training at this institution, however the positive thing that was revealed during the test was that it revealed incredible increases in fat burning potential in just seven exercise sessions. That's the exaggeration of the HIIT training. In any case, I'm going to keep you in mind for a different test that was conducted during the course of McMaster University , Ontario in the year 2006. I'm thinking there's some kind of competition between the Ontario institutions to become the experts in HIIT ask about. 16 people were randomly tossed out to either an HIIT group or one of the CT group.

Each group took part in 6 educational meetings over the course of 14 days on bikes. The HIIT group was involved in four to six 30-second , full-scale intervals of exercise and 4 moments of recuperation between. The CT group participated in 90-120-minute sessions with a 70% of their maximum heart rate. The muscle biopsy tests were performed after the test has shown that there was a similar increase in carbohydrate oxidative capacities in both groups. But, if you think about it again, what is the difference between the above test? Take a look at the general exercise definitions for both groups, as the differences here are huge in actual fact.

The HIIT group practice sessions lasted for an average of 22.5 minutes, compared to the CT group that ran for more than 105 minutes. In the course of the study it was 2 hours and 15 minutes (HIIT) and 10 hours 30 minutes (CT). That's it. With only a tiny fraction of the exercise duration, HIIT is practically identical to CT in regards to enhancing the muscle mass and the capacity to oxidize carbohydrate.

Abundance Post Exercise Oxygen Consumption (EPOC)

The other system I referred to is called oxygen obligation, also known as overabundance post-practice oxygen usage (EPOC). If you've read a large quantity on health and well-being and health, you might see EPOC described as the after consumption impact.

When you train at full intensity, like you would in an HIIT session the oxygen-consuming framework will not in any way, form or manner provide you with the necessary energy to power the exercise. Although it'll perform with a great effort and offer all you that it can it, the anaerobic framework isn't going to have any choice other than to be an integral part of the process to provide extra vitality assistance. The most common time this point is between 65 and 85 percent of your maximum heart rate, which is what we'll explore in the next section. I'll clarify the rules of EPOC by using an illustration. Imagine going for a swim from one end of a lake and then the next. You realize that it will take about an hour to complete the swim, so typically you decide to take your time.

Whatever your goal to reach the other side of the lake within as fast as you could be allowed, you'd at your current pace so that you don't run out in energy too soon. But, imagine a situation when a shark suddenly appeared and started to swim towards you. You are fortunate to see an immense rock right in front of you, just a few minute's swim away. So you go full-throttle and do everything you have to do to get to the rock and save your life. In the present, do you think you'd inhale more strongly upon reaching the rock, or after arriving on the other part of the lake? Naturally, the correct reaction is to breathe more forcefully after reaching the rock. This is because switching on the burners to full has put an enormous and rapid weight on your digestion process that uses oxygen and this is mainly the reason that you're breathing so intensely. One of the most fundamental aspects of development and physiological principle will be that the body adapts to the pressure.

Therefore, in the unlikely possibility that you are able to escape sharks constantly or, even better, you can impersonate the shark in a more controlled setting such as in a pool, then your body will increase. Another reason you're now breathing more deeply when you reach the rock, as opposed to when you reach the bottom of the lake, is because the moment you arrive, you require more oxygen to replenish your vital reserves of energy that were used in scurry by the non-oxidative pathways of metabolism (see Energy Systems underneath) to keep you safe from sharks.

The current situation is crucial and you'll need to control the astonishingly amount of lactic acid that has formed in your muscles in the course of the swim due to increasing the speed to maximum. The growth of lactic acid had no relation to the swimming itself however it's there because of the intense nature of the swimmingafter being able to escape the shark. The increased oxygen consumption, which is expected to continue for several hours, will continue creating a reaction in the body. This is what is meant by the phrase EPOC or the after-consumption effect. After you have finished the procedure of making, however, you're still consuming energy or calories at an increased rate due to the intensity of the task.

It is important to stress that there isn't any EPOC from CT since the activity just not escalated enough. EPOC is simply increased after the high intensity activity. How long will EPOC continue to increase? This is dependent on the seriousness of the event. The more severe the event The more prominent the EPOC. The effects of EPOC is the highest during the first couple of hours after practice, in the time when the body is in the greatest need to recover. The impact of EPOC is then gradual decreases over the next 48 hours. The more intense earlier exercise is, the greater EPOC continues to occur.

Energy Systems

Each system makes use of starch and fat for fuel at different frequencies. Each system operates to different amounts based on degree of activity. They're working constantly in the dark and are able to slide throughout the activity based on the task at hand. This ATP system is employed in high-intensity activities like running and lasts for the longest time for about 10 seconds or less prior to becoming exhausted. The word ATP refers to adenosine triphosphate that is found in a limited reserves in our bodies but don't be concerned when you run out of it, your body will quickly make it back, which is a blessing for those who HIIT typically. The glycogen/lactic acid system can go for an extended period than from 30 seconds to three minutes or more, based on your fitness.

Glycogen is your body's supply of energy that it uses to do everything. It generally will be available. It is what that we use for the majority times, especially when we're eating, sleeping or watching TV or engaging in light-to-direct exercises. When we exercise CT for extended periods the body is using one energy system, it's called the aerobic system. When we reach the 65-85percent of the max range of pulses (depending on the degree of fitness) is the glycogen system emerge as the most significant factor. This is where you are actually making use of energy in two different ways. This is where that we must aim to reach (or significantly higher) but only for short time when participating during the HIIT program. It's true that in HIIT it is best to aim to 100percent of the maximum pulse to help build up our ATP system, too. In this way, we're utilizing energy on three different levels. Not just two and not just one.

Contrary to CT, HIIT gives a exercise to all three of the energy systems, not just those in the aerobic. It gives us a more effective workout, and comes with numerous physical advantages for us which a dull CT session cannot match. Through participating in HIIT it will give you significant increases in the post-exercise fat burning, beyond the benefits CT can provide. It is best to think of this as a free time for training as you've finished your exercise session, however your body still burns fat at a higher rate. To help clarify this further I'll give you a reference to the results of a study which showed that for 24 hours following the conclusion of a HIIT workout, HIIT subjects were still burning calories at a high rate, while CT subjects did not. For the course of 24 hours following sessions with HIIT, this was equivalent to an additional 100 calories burned compared to that of the CT group. This is a significant figure and explains why HIIT participants are able to get more energy out of themselves and shed more fat while doing the same amount of work as CT participants.

To better understand the reason you burn fat at a high rate after HIIT exercises, I'll be referring to another study which was conducted within Laval University in Quebec in 1994. The research was conducted to study the impact from CT or HIIT on body fat and the metabolism of muscles. 32 participants were randomly assigned to the CT group or one of the HIIT groups. The CT group was part of 20 weeks of training, while the HIIT group was part of the course of 15 weeks. When the study was over protocol, the estimated mean energy cost for those in the CT group stood at 120.4 MJ, while the average estimated energy expense of those in the HIIT group was 57.9 J. Consider that these numbers are based on the energy costs incurred of the exercise routine alone and not the addition of EPOC. Take into consideration how it was the CT group's exercise regimen ran for 5 weeks more than those in the HIIT group. This isn't the way I would have planned for the research, however let's just go on this.

Then, at the conclusion of the study, measurement was taken on the skinfolds and the HIIT group was observed to have experienced an increase in body fat nine times higher than CT. CT group. Reread that. Nine times more! This is despite the fact that the amount of energy consumed in the exercise routine was over two times higher within the CT group than that of the HIIT group. The only way this could be explained is the fact that there are an energy-saving physiological change taking place after exercise, which produces large quantities of lactate (HIIT).

It also proves that it's not all about the length of time spent exercising however, it's the degree of the exercise. I'm sure you've heard about the phrase "no pain, no gain" that was invented by Benjamin Franklin. It's a fact.

Anaerobic Threshold

What is the anaerobic threshold? to? It's the time that you transition into the aerobic into glycogen/lactic acid systems. If you exercise at any intensity, lactic acid begins to build up in bloodstreams. The greater intensities, the quicker it accumulates. The intensity of exercise is increased to the point that it is producing lactic acid greater than the rate at which it is removed in blood. It eventually builds to a higher level that causes discomfort. This is known as the threshold for anaerobic exercise. In reality the moment you exercise, it's the moment at which the pain, performance that prevents the building-up of lactic acid is felt in muscles. In general, in non-trained athletes the anaerobic threshold is likely to be about 65% of maximum heart rate. The healthier the person then the higher their anaerobic threshold. So if we carry out CT work, we will rarely cross the threshold for anaerobic activity. What are the implications of this?

This means that you won't being training different energy system. If we are crossing the threshold of anaerobic activity repeatedly, like during HIIT it is a constant training of the anaerobic energy system (glycogen/lactic acid system as well as the ATP system). What effect can this affect us? Since we're creating more lactic acids in our muscles and organs, our bodies will need to adjust to this. Within a short period of time our anaerobic threshold is pushed back. Instead of feeling the uncomfortable lactic acid build-up around the 65% mark of your maximum heart rate, you'll experiencing it at 70 percent of your maximum then 75%, and then percent. What's happening is that your body is getting more effective at tackling the painful build-up of lactic acid and allowing you to put in more effort and longer without feeling the burning sensation.

If you increase your anaerobic threshold, in essence, you are improving your aerobic performance because the amount of work that you can perform aerobically has increased in relation to anaerobic activity. In actual terms how has this had on your health and function? A higher endurance can benefit your life in a variety of ways, especially if you had previously been unconditioned. There is no reason to feel exhausted while doing your day-to-day routine. You will no longer feel an increase in the acid lactic from participating in any painful physical exercise.

Do you imagine how this could increase the health of people? It will be possible to go for walks in the countryside when you're on vacation, and spend time with your children and not break an ice. If grocery shopping is, for instance, at times a struggle for you, you'll be able to complete this task without feeling of exhaustion that you experienced prior to. This is just one of the benefits of training that comes from HIIT. We're becoming more fit by achieving levels that CT cannot achieve. HIIT enhances our ability to tolerate ever-increasing intensity exercises. This is the reason professional athletes like Footballers are often trained using HIIT as it can help delay the production of lactic acid, which causes fatigue. It is a great benefit for athletes who play sports in which there is a constant changing of the pace, like Football, Rugby, Badminton and Tennis, which is nearly all of sports currently played.

Anaerobic Capacity

Anaerobic threshold refers to the extent of work that could be done prior to reaching the glycogen/lactic corrosive framework anaerobic capability refers to the amount of work that is done using both glycogen/lactic corrosive as well as ATP frameworks. It's the quantity of work that could be completed between the first sensation of discomfort and then stepping out of a store on the ground. I'll now show how simple it is to plan your workouts and making significant gains, citing an famous study conducted by an Japanese scientist whose name might recognize.

In 1996 in 1996, in 1996, Dr. Izumi Tabata structured a study aimed at discovering what effects CT or HIIT (actually Tabata) on anaerobic capacity. By using a cycle ergometer subjects trained five days a week for approximately 1 month and half. The CT group worked for one hour at a 70% maximum heart rate. The HIIT group was working in 20 second increments at 100% intensity, with a 10 second in rest, for a total of eight sessions. The time to complete the HIIT exercise was just 4 minutes. After the conclusion of the study participants in the CT group was not found to have experienced significant increases in their anaerobic capacity. This isn't surprising given that those who were in an unbeatable 70% max heart rate are likely not to be able to pass the threshold of anaerobic fitness. The HIIT group had nevertheless experienced increases of 28% to anaerobic capacity.

It's from exercises that last just four minutes. While reading this text, you could consider that it's perfectly fine, however I seldom need to train until I am done. This is why I say that you should never face an emergency situation where you have to live through life as if your life, or that of a loved one or family member was dependent on it. But, an increase in anaerobic power should be considered as an extra benefit for any expert or leisure athlete who usually exceeds the threshold for anaerobic fitness. Much like HIIT itself, Tabata is a kind of HIIT is becoming increasingly popular all over the world.

BetaEndorphin Levels

Beta-endorphin can be described as the "vibe fantastic" element that's accountable for the reason we often feel after a intense exercise. It's created in the cerebrum's nerve center as a reaction to pain. If we experience pain, physical or emotional the brain is eventually de-sensitized due to the release of beta-endorphin. The beta-endorphin components are diverse and serve as pain relieving and bringing us a feeling of joy is the fact that it's believed to reduce the growth of cancer cells, and can allow us to relax as well. Because beta-endorphin develops when we feel relief from pain and we can see that large amounts are infused during strenuous exercise like HIIT, for instance. This is due to the pain of lactic acid which develops in our muscles. The beta-endorphin tries to ease the pain.

In other words, when we simply exercise CT workouts, beta-endorphin won't be generated in the same manner. The truth is: "Distributed investigations uncover that periodic review and a momentary exercise result in an increase in beta-endorphin levelsto in a manner that is linked to lactate concentration." Naturally, when we say "anaerobic" it refers to an ongoing, intense exercise, such as HIIT. The study revealed that a greater amount of beta-endorphin will be released when you are working out harder because you'll produce more an increase in lactic acid and beta-endorphin will be produced as a response to this. The study also went on to prove that levels of beta-endorphin do not increase when exercising in a continuous level, as is the case using CT in the event that the CT is prolonged for more than 60 mins.

This could help clarify what is known as the "sprinters high" sensation that is often reported by long-distance sprinters. The main goal in this section is to illustrate how the "vibe wonderful" substance that influences our minds-sets is more effectively created through the combination of a HIIT exercise over an CT exercise and how by training in intervals with high intensity, you're creating the conditions for a full day of high-energy state. It's for a long time been believed that exercise induces positive emotions, induces a sense of excitement and can also be an effective remedy for sadness, however the link between the force of exercise and your emotions is not widely established.

Maximal Oxygen Uptake/VO2 Max

It's the person's VO2 max, which is frequently utilized to calculate their fitness level overall. The fitness of your cardio-respiratory system is measured by the amount of oxygen consumed, which is called VO2 according to the American College of Sports Medicine (ACSM). The "V" refers to Volume, while "O2" obviously refers to oxygen. This is deliberate because it's an approximate rate for oxygen consumption in milliliters per kg of weight per minutes (ml/kg/min). The term VO2 max refers to the ability of an individual to utilize and store oxygen throughout the course of their activity. When we train in a way that gets more intense the limit increases because our lungs and hearts are progressively efficient in transferring oxygen-rich blood to muscles, which in turn improve their effectiveness in using the oxygen. Therefore, we must look at the results of a few studies that evaluate and compare HIIT and CT to the VO2 max.

A study found that 27 heart dissatisfaction patients with an average age of 75 were in HIIT as well as CT group. The HIIT group trained at the rate at 95% maximum heart rate. The CT group worked at 70 percent. The sessions were held 3 times per every week over 12 weeks. the VO2 max was measured at the beginning and at the close in the course of study. After 12 weeks the HIIT group increased their maximum VO2 by 46% whereas the CT group only increased their VO2 max by 14 percent. This is an amazing result for HIIT.

In a separate study, 25 men, with a mean time of 10 years were randomized in either an HIIT or the CT group. The CT group exercised for 20 minutes each session with 80 to 85 percent of their maximum heart rate. The HIIT group ran 30-second bursts on a stationary cycling cycle, which were followed with recuperation intervals for 20 minutes. Vo2max was measured towards the beginning and at the close of the three-week study. At the conclusion this study two groups saw an increase in the VO2 max. The HIIT class being the clear champion. This is it. In terms of improving your general fitness according to the VO2 max, which is the best measure of fitness in general ever created the HIIT method is superior to CT.

What other details did you observe about the two researches mentioned that you mentioned above? The first study was conducted with patients suffering from heart problems one of them was 86 years old. In the second research, subjects were young children. The two tests required strenuous exercises at more than 95 percent of their heart rate at their highest. The results of these tests show that HIIT, despite being extremely active, is a sure-fire safe workout and even energizes any person, regardless of their age or fitness.Have you ever thought about getting tested for your personal maximum VO2? There are many ways to do it.

The most straightforward method is to use a treadmill or stationary bicycle in the rec center (in case you're a resident who is a member of one).

Typically, you'll be ready for a few minutes and then walk, run or cycle in a frenzied manner, overcoming obstacles or angles, until you are unable to do it again. Because the goal is to determine the highest amount of oxygen that your body can absorb into, you'll be pushed to the maximum extent possible (be advised) and, now, the duration you ran until you finish is recorded. The time is then placed into a state, focusing of the gender of your body (just as old age and other variables based on the condition used). Then, you will receive an exact number, which is your VO2 maximum (in milliliters oxygen/kg bodyweight) per second (ml/kg/min). Based on this figure, you can evaluate it against the norms for your gender and age in the event you choose to. If you do, then more important, keep an account of your scores and use it as a guideline for your VO2 max tests in the future. I am confident that if you do regular HIIT sessions that your VO2 max will grow at a steady rate.

Athletic Performance

What sports require lengthy periods of continuous exercise? There are some, but not all of them; distance swimming, distance running distance cycling, distance rowing. If you consider it, almost all sports require stopping and beginning an action. From combat sports, like boxing and martial art, racket sports, such as squash and tennis up to team sports like football as well as American and soccer, as and basketball as well as hockey on ice. Additionally, there are the track and field sports, like jumping, both high and long shooting, shot putting or any other throwing event, and of course, there's sprinting as well. All these sports because of short bursts in high-intensity activities will trigger the rapid production of the acid lactic.

In this regard, managing this challenging performance damaging lactic acid is crucial for all athletes or for the casual sportsperson. If you aren't able to handle focus on high lactate then you'll face an enormous disadvantage when compared against any competitor who is prepared for HIIT. Furthermore, you will not be able to compete with your opponents will not be the only thing to worry about - you'll be battling any person who's competing in the exact scenario as you do on the team for games such as your team. For everything in life, if you feel you have to become proficient in something, then you need to practice the skill. In case, in your sports, you need to manage large clusters of acid lactic when you need to put in order for your body to be proficient at removing it, you're likely have to produce tons of it.

Your body will soon discover the best way to manage the lactic acid. You will adapt as a result. In the meantime you should be informed of the fact that HIIT is the most effective method for causing this build-up of lactic acid. As of now you won't be astonished to discover that your ability to combat build-ups of lactic acid can be achieved quickly by participating the HIIT. One study has proven that just six sessions of HIIT over 14 days could effectively reduce the build-up of lactic acid within the legs following high-force cycling.

The HIIT Diving into

A WRARM-UP STRETCH AS WELL COOLDOWN

It is important to always get your body ready by warming up prior to every workout. The reason for this is that it helps prevent any wounds caused by viruses because when they're cold, they're less malleable. This means they're more tightly packed and will offer limited amount of room for growth. As muscles get warmed up, they will become more flexible and less prone to wounds that are caused by reason and become more flexible. This means that you can enjoy the fullest potential for development. It means that exercise becomes easier to perform, and you'll be able to enjoy an increasingly enjoyable exercise.

The most efficient way to WARM-UPis

If you're participating in any of my high-intensity indoor exercises then you're left with two options. You can start your march for a few minutes, and then after an increment in height of your legs while you walk and arc your arms to your sides. On the other hand you could march through the steps for a few minutes. In the event that you're doing one of my HIIT open-air exercises and you are there you could simply walk at a steady pace for about two minutes. After you've warmed-up it's an excellent idea to stretch the major muscles. It is also an essential thing to perform towards the end of your workout as it allows the muscles to heal and prevents irritation to muscles.

Calf Stretch

Move back on one leg. Keep your back leg straight and the point of impact down with your two feet facing towards the forward direction. Bend your knee on the leg in front, and feel your palms on your bent leg. Feel the stretch in your lower leg as it is stretched back behind. Ten seconds is the time to warm up, and 15 seconds to cool down.

Hamstring Stretch

Place one leg in front, place the heel on the floor , and then twist your knee on the leg in the back. Then, place two hands on the back side and stretch all the way across to the rear of your straight leg. Keep it for 10 seconds to warm up and 20 seconds to cool down.

Quadriceps Stretch

Keep your posture straight and then twist the leg behind you. Bring your foot towards the cheek of the butt. Hold the foot with care or sock of your bent leg. Maintain the knee that is supporting it bent. Keep it bent for 10 seconds on each leg for your warm-up, and then at least 15 seconds each leg for cooling down.

Triceps Stretch

Keep a solid straight back, firm and straight and knees bent slightly and your stomach pulled in. Take one arm and bend it around your head with the intention to put your hand in into the shoulder bone. Make sure to support it carefully with the other arm. As you warm-up you should hold it for 10 seconds. At that time, repeat the exercise with the second arm. Do 15 seconds of hold on each arm to allow for a cooling down.

Chest Stretch

Maintain your posture with good posture and keep your arms in front of you. You can lift your shoulders back and up so that you feel your chest stretch. your chest. Do this for 10 seconds to complete your warm-up. You should hold for 15 seconds for your cooling down.

Back Stretch

Maintain a good posture. Keep your knees in a comfortable position and keep your keep your tummy into. Keep your arms out in the front of you and imagine you're embracing a massive volleyball. Feel the stretch in your back. Ten seconds of holding is your warm-up. You should hold for 15 seconds for your cooling down.

Health and Safety

This is among the most important topics to study in this book, since your security and well-being is the most important aspect, and you should adhere to these rules while working out.

You should always:

*Warm up, stretch, and then relax as a key part of your exercise.

Listen to your body and in the event something hurts or feels not right, take a break.

Drink lots of water.

*If you're outside you are, then apply sunscreen and stay away from the dawn sun.

If you're outside, make sure to take your cell phone and constantly inform someone where you're headed.

If outside, dress in sparkling clothing.

What's more, Never:

Do some exercise if you're experiencing a feeling of sickness.

Feel a little agitated following an injury and get back to training and be patient, because it could pay dividends over the long term.

* Work out with a empty stomach.

*Do exercises that cause pain.

Also, the most important thing is to Do not be afraid to ask questions and Find the time to complete one of these workouts.

In the event that you cause injury to yourself.

The first thing you need do on the off possibility of injuring yourself during your practice is stop immediately! It is recommended for bruises, injuries, sprains or swelling to apply ice treatment immediately on the site where the injury occurred.

Ice therapy is the best treatment on a fresh injury. When we are injured the bloodstream increases towards the affected area because this is the body's first step in fixing the injury. The influx of blood is a great way to irritate nerves and in turn causes painful swelling. If swelling isn't managed it could cause tissue damage further, which is why it should be reduced. The benefits of applying ice are to reduce the amount of blood that flows into tissues, lessen or prevent swelling (aggravation) and reduce the muscle pain and fits and ease pain by reducing the sensitivity of the region and restricting the effects of swelling. TheradegPEARL ice packs are available through www.therapearl.com.

The effects of reducing swelling help to prevent the region from becoming solid due to the reduction of tissue liquids that build up because of the aggravation and injury. It doesn't matter if it's ruptured tendon, bruising muscle soreness, or bruising. Ice packs can be effective in transferring them into the cooler , and then after it is applied, they protect your body from repeated injury and permanent harm. If you're preparing for your next appointment, bring a THERAdegPEARL pack in the event of an unexpected issue. And, interestingly it conforms to your body, so that it can be applied pressure to the affected area easily. Always apply ice for 20 minutes. You should do not apply ice treatment on areas of the skin that have low sensation of temperatures or chills, or on regions of your body that have a an established poor condition in the case of diabetes, or in the proximity of any contamination. Make sure you allow for a complete recovery from any injury prior to you return to exercise. Although it's not ideal, it's worth a moment of pause for a while, you may end getting worsening an injury and it's an excellent idea to have the injury evaluated by a medical professional or expert.

Workout INTENSITY GUIDE

It is crucial to work out at a predetermined level of power to reap the benefits of high intensity training.

The process of measuring the power of your workout can be difficult cost-intensive, as well as tedious however, you can discover and alter one of the most important information about the world of wellness the RATE OF EXERTION PERCEIVED. This RPE scale lets you determine the power level you're preparing for to ensure that you are able to be sure that you're working with the correct force to perform the HIIT exercises.

I recommend to familiarize yourself with this scale since we reference this scale throughout our book and every workout will list the RPE level you need to be training at.

1. Absolutely nothing (sitting on the couch)

2. Very Light, extremely

3. Extremely light (gentle exercises)

4. Moderate

5. A bit difficult

6. It's hard (unable to engage in an ongoing conversation)

7. Very difficult

8. Very, very difficult

9. Near exhaustion

10. Maximum

Chapter 8: Training For Hiit

The purpose of this chapter is to intention is to open your mind to the various choices available to you should you be keen to give HIIT a go. Therefore, we will outline the exercises in detail and proceed to HIIT cycling which will be the main focus of the next chapter of this book.

Sprinting

Sprinting has been shown to be a successful method to conduct high-intensity interval training. It involves intervals of fast speed running, followed by shorter periods of walking , or taking complete breaks. I typically do not suggest anyone who is not at their best for this type of workout since they are at risk of injury. Even those who are confident of their fitness level there are rules to be followed during this exercise.

The process begins by heading to a track and giving yourself go. Begin by warming up, before taking the 20 second sprint. Then, follow it up with a 10 seconds of jumping, and then take a 30 second break or walk. The exercise has been proven to be extremely efficient in burning off calories.

Push-Ups

The push-ups are a great way to build your muscles and strengthening them. In order to do this it is necessary to perform at minimum 30 push-ups or press-ups without taking a break. Then you'll have to follow it with low-intensity exercise that allows your body to recover. it is possible to follow this exercise with a full relaxation. Here's how you accomplish this:

1. Put yourself into a plank position, placing your hands on the floor as they sit directly beneath your shoulders. Your legs should be at least the same width.

2. Bend your elbows and your entire body until your body is touching the ground, keeping your elbows resting against your sides, and your body is in straight lines. Go as low as you can before returning to the starting position and continue the workout 30 times.

Squat jumps

For this workout, squat then make a small leap ahead and then return to your squat. Repeat the exercise at least 45 times , and then follow it up by doing a slow-intensity exercise so that your body can recover. If you enjoy this exercise, make sure you do it frequently as it may cause certain post-effects on your muscles which can cause pain if not utilized regularly.

Sit-ups

1. For this, start by lying on your back, with your knees bent and your feet are placed on the floor. Once you have tightened the core, then you can pull your head back using your abs. Then lift your head back to the floor until you're actually standing up straight while your back is parallel to the floor.

2. Relax slowly and engage your abs. Then, return to your starting position. You can then repeat your exercise fifty times.

Tricep Dip

Begin by stepping onto all fours as you look towards the ceiling while knees bent 90 degrees, right over your toes. Your hands are positioned just below your shoulders. When you are done the fingers must be facing upwards and the back of your body is straight, so the core of your body is in line with the ground.

Relax your elbows as they are folded in such that your butt is as far as you are able to. Then, push up and repeat the exercise for 10 times.

Other HIIT exercises you can attempt include split jumps burpees and jump squats to name some. While there are many more exercises that can be done with HIIT however, the primary goal is to make sure you burn off fat for throughout the day after your workout. For this to be accomplished with greater ease, it's ideal to consider the HIIT bike to help you burn more calories and reap all the benefits associated from high intensity training. We will go over HIIT biking in the following chapters.

Bicycle Training for HIIT for Effective HIIT Exercise

In the preceding chapter, we discussed various workouts can be utilized to increase your intensity during interval training. I intentionally left out cycling as we devote this book to learning to successfully do it. Numerous professionals suggest cycling to those looking to speed up their pace at the track. They also recommend that you shed weight and build their muscles, to name some of the benefits you will gain from HIIT cycling training.

Why do we need to HIIT cycling?

Numerous studies have proven bike training's legitimacy as the most effective method of getting the most results HIIT. Here's why you should consider HIIT training.

The fats component

It is a fact biking on the bike is more energy-efficient than other types of exercise. Furthermore, you'll burn calories even when you are when you are not exercising. If you force your body to boost its metabolism and burn stored fat to satisfy energy needs. It is essential that your diet be low in calories so that your body is able to reach a energy deficit, to allow it to use stored fat to generate energy.

If your aim is to push your body to shed fat You should be performing high-intensity riding (I will demonstrate how to do this later in the book).

Additionally, biking can increase the threshold for lactate (that threshold at which your legs begin to hurt like a bee and you have only one option: slow down) which makes you a high-calorie eater. This means you'll be burning lots of calories, even after you have exercised.

The speed factor

The intensity of your riding can raise the threshold for lactate and VOX2Max. The intensity of your riding will increase the amount of oxygen consumed to its maximum (VOX2Max). If you are a heavy oxygen user, you build a strong cardiovascular system that can provide a sufficient flow with oxygen rich blood. This allows for a smooth coordination with your muscle and the nerve system, which improves your speed and endurance.

The lactate threshold is the threshold at which your legs begin to hurt like an insect bite, and you have only one option: slow down. The intervals will increase the threshold of lactate so that you change into a faster rider with a high endurance.

The energy factor

The energy we need comes from an energised body that is well-supplied with oxygen and blood, coupled with a good nerve coordination. This is exactly what cycling involves. The muscles we use also get stronger as we add more stress to them. Therefore, if you're cycling regularly then you don't have to perform a second session to build up your muscles.

So, now that we know the basics of what HIIT cycling on bikes is about Let's narrow it down to the particular HIIT cycling strategies you should use.

An indoor cycling jumps

This workout can be completed outdoors or indoors on roads. While your hands are firmly on the handlebars your body with your hips to the side and then forward over the bike's seat and then back to the upright posture. After you've achieved this posture, you can hold your position and jump each time.

The swaying motion, when combined with the effort you use to balance and hold your bike grip creates a fantastic muscle tone. Dr. Tabata suggests that you could integrate this exercise into your music. How?

He suggests that you opt to do sets of, say, 10 for these workouts. Then, allow the beats of the music to guide your movement forward and backwards as you perform the jumping exercises. Then, he claims, it will eliminate boredom. Since this is high intensity interval training, it is recommended to take a minute break after performing 10 sets of jumping. This will allow your muscles to recover.

You can also switch sets of standing and sitting jumps for maximum fat burnout. Always aim to get the the most control on your bicycle by increasing the resistance. Bike jumps are perfect for generating maximum impact on your muscles. They also have the effect of strengthening their muscles. It's also a great method to burn calories.

Interval hill sprints

Similar to normal sprints toward the hills, the resistance is more intense when you climb the hill when riding, rather than riding on flat surfaces. It tests the strength and strength of the legs.

In order to do this exercise on the bike begin by lowering the resistance first and let your leg go through as many turns per minute as feasible. Take a moment to get out of your seat in intervals of 5 seconds each to completely engage your body in the workout. Make sure that your hips are in a uniform movement together with your legs. The aim is to make every muscle part of your body take part in the exercise , allowing the maximum burning of calories.

Start with the first 10 seconds of this exercise to increase your speed and then the following ten seconds to maintain that momentum. At the end of each race, you should allow you to take between one and two minutes to rest. A leisurely cycling, perhaps on an even surface is good.

But, if you're performing it for the very first time you should not push yourself too hard

Start slowly and gradually increase the speed until you're physically fit enough to perform the exercise the way pros do it.

Tabata cycling

Dr. Tabata has come out with a method that is considered to be the most efficient cardio exercises by a lot of experts since it delivers more significant results than standard aerobic exercises.

It involves 20 second workouts with a rest of 10 seconds. For the duration of period of 20 minutes, Tabata recommends to sprint, i.e. cycle, at least the speed of between 80 and 90% that of the maximum rate. This should be your highest intensity training interval. After 20 seconds, reduce your speed to minimum 60 percent at your highest speed in order to enable recovery.

Try to complete minimum 8 or 12 cycles of Tabata that are repeated and help reduce fat faster than you normally do! This type of fitness has gained a lot of popularity as the most sought-after high-intensity training. It's also possibly among the more intense exercises. It is extremely effective in building muscle, improving strength and fitness, and losing fat. Amazingly, it's the most efficient workout.

Perform your 8-12 intervals, then continue with your other activities. The effects last for several hours.

Sitting in a hazy position

While your hands are firmly placed on the bars, shift your hips forward and you will find your butt practically hovering over your seat by 3 inches. Stay in this position for about 45 minutes. Repeat the exercise for 1 to 3 times in addition to your regular exercise routine. If you are able to accomplish it while biking simultaneously then you're doing it right.

There are some who don't know what to do with their hamstrings during exercises like cycling. This workout is the most effective for you if you're one. It gives a high-intensity sensation to your quads and hamstrings. Make sure you don't grip the handlebars too tightly. Give it a gentle gesture, while allowing you to the ability to control your bike.

I'm sure you've learned about other exercises that you were not aware of the HIIT bike workout program. In the next section we'll shift our attention on the preparations needed for this exercise.

Training Plans For Cyclists

Recently, I attended an event where one of the participants asked me to present them with a an example of a plan they could apply to their HIIT bicycle training program. I was caught off guard, and I promised him that I would write it down in this instructional.

While you've been learning about HIIT I'm sure you are aware that the more you push yourself in a given time, the better you become at it. This is more difficult to achieve in the absence of an action strategy. Therefore, a exercise plan can be your difference when it comes to success or failing when it comes to high intensity training. Simply put, make a plan for your ride and become more proficient at. If you're looking to be a better cyclist then you shouldn't wake up and start riding randomly.

The planning of your workouts demands understanding the energy used during each exercise. This article will explore the role of different energy systems to every exercise (these depend on the length of time the exercise occurs). The body's energy use is described in the three systems of energy: glycolytic, aerobic and the ATP system. The extent to which each is utilized is based on the length and intensity of each exercise:

1. ATP is the main ingredient responsible for instantaneous energy. It utilizes adenosinetriphosphate (ATP) to create this energy. This is what makes us sprint. within our bodies. It produces this energy for a couple of glorious seconds when it breaks the ATP chemically and providing an instant surge of energy. ATP energy can only last between 10 and 30 seconds. When this energy has gone it is imperative to allow your body the time to replenish its supply of ATP. This is where the recovery time during your workouts is crucial.

2. The glycolytic system, also known as the anaerobic system , lasts longer than ATP system. It's not as demanding. You can exercise your muscles for between 2 and 10

128

minutes with an anaerobic process. The system converts glycogen to lactic acid , which helps regenerate muscle cells that are oxygen-deficient. It's the energy that keeps you going after a run or climb.

3. The second body system that is involved in aerobics. It is the one responsible for the energy that drives long mountain climb. It is through this system that blood provides oxygen to muscles of the body. This oxygen is used to breakdown glycogen into carbon dioxide. This creates a sustainable source of energy source for your pedals. Aerobic system is what powers behind long rides that last more than 5 minutes or less.

When you do HIIT cycling exercises, the objective is to strengthen the cardiovascular system in order that it will last longer. What is the best way to do get there? Here's how:

Step 1: Begin by strengthening your strength

Muscles are often the weakest link for all riders. The reason isn't that the muscles are weak, but that they release too fast. If you feel exhausted, and it originates from your leg muscles, your training plan is over regardless of the reason. To avoid this issue I suggest you target around 60 percent of the max for a period of 2 weeks, based on the duration you intend to exercise. It should be continued until your muscles have become used to the strain. This is essential due to the fact that muscles other than the lungs and heart don't recover as fast. This type of low-intensity exercise is , therefore, extremely beneficial.

Step 2: Change into stronger cycling

Once you've built your muscles up and stronger, it's time to begin to intensify your training. The first step is getting to the aerobic threshold. The threshold is where your body begins to go into an oxygen deficit, however you are able to maintain the state for minimum 30 minutes if the situation demands. If you are able to maintain this state for more than 30 minutes, you're not trying at all as hard as I'd like that you will be. If you can't keep it for more than 15 minutes, then congratulations and congratulations! You've done well!

It is crucial to be able to discern your threshold. It is easy to determine the threshold point by doing an uphill sprint on your bike, and recording your number of revolutions in a minutes (rpm) up to the point where you feel the rhythm of your breathing change.

The most important thing to make this part of the beginning of your HIIT cycle training program is to ensure that there is sufficient tension on your muscles throughout the entire time. Making sure you are pedaling in a consistent manner while keeping your upper body still is another key to success.

This phase should be completed at least two or 3 intervals during each workout , and then followed by 10 minutes recovery time.

Step 3: Dissolving the pedal stroke

This should be at the highest level of your fitness I suggest to use the highest gear. This will enable you to accelerate, sit on your bike and hang onto the bike until you are at the finish line without needing to change gears.

Make a smooth and steady acceleration, and then return to the saddle and making sure that you don't fail to make any pedal stroke. You may choose to have the beginning point and an end point that gives 30 seconds for recovery between.

Because this stage is more advanced, six intervals for each workout are sufficient. A recovery time of 5 minutes is acceptable.

Step 4 4. High spin

It is possible to do this with simple or comfortable equipment. This doesn't require you to go uphill or use a raised surface. Flat surfaces will work perfectly.

If you're a beginner (of course, form is of paramount importance as well) Start at 100rpm , then increase it to at least 130 rotations per minute. Don't be concerned when your heart rate is reaching the aerobic threshold in a short amount of time. Since you've worked on strengthening your body during the final stages, it is able to adapt to this shift.

I don't wish for your speed to reach prior to the limit, therefore, we'll only allow the duration to 10 minutes, followed by an recovery. Because it is easy to achieve, you can perform it in recuperation time or on days.

While you have the essential workout phases you must follow but it could be insufficient if I fail in preparing you to perform this important exercise. Every workout should start with a 20 minute warm up, however I suggest that should there is more time it is possible to do a 30-40 minutes of warming up to prepare yourself for the job. It shouldn't be a problem in the event that you are mentally prepared for the task.

Another thing to remember is that you must never neglect your recovery time. Don't allow your trainers to stress you more than is necessary. The recovery period is equally important as that of the actual training.

It is easy to adjust to your exercise routine. It also allows the body to re-energize its capabilities and systems, allowing you to be more prepared for the next task.

Recovery and rest are beneficial in recovering energy and healing tissues and muscles, which allows you to be more efficient in the following exercise because you will be able to adapt your body's structure to that requirements of the activity.

Improves endurance in aerobic. If you take a break or go to recover, you improve the endurance of your aerobic system or to provide adequate oxygen supply so you are able to endure difficult and tiring physical exercise.

In simple terms When you perform high intensity workouts that push your body to produce a metabolic need that aids in long-term weight loss and general conditioning and rest (low intensity intervals) between them helps to recover , and possibly utilize an aerobic energy system.

Note:

It is not necessary to make this exercise interrupt your regular routines. It is possible to continue riding longer bursts of speed and still burn a lot of calories into your body. Your plan should not have to be different from the ones you'll find on the numerous websites you visit. Take a look at the time to work with and then plan your time based on your own personal obligations. The reason for this is that recovery time is essential in your HIIT bike workout routines.

Notice: Different bicycles utilize different strategies to accomplish their objectives. But, they aren't that distinct in their fundamentals.

It's easy to think that HIIT cycling is an exercise that gives you every benefit. It's not as simple as that. You have to participate in a variety of types of HIIT cycling in order to reap the many benefits that come from HIIT cycling. Let's examine these in the following chapter.

HIIT Bicycle Training Courses

In the earlier sections we believed that the strategy is the same for each exercise session, regardless of whether the goal is endurance, speed improvement and fat reduction. This was a mistake, though it was supposed to help explain the issues we were discussing in the moment. There are a variety of disciplines that are associated with biking and it's crucial to know the best discipline for each scenario. Each discipline require a distinct training regimen. This section will we'll shift our attention to a subset particular disciplines.

Road racing

The cyclists in this group are believed to have a lot of endurance. A number of studies have revealed an aerobic strength high among this group of cyclists. A majority of people who participate in the program have been athletes that want to improve their speed.

A measure called lactate threshold is used extensively within this system to assess the performance. The lactate threshold is the threshold where your legs begin to hurt, causing you to reduce your speed. Training intervals is said to raise your lactate threshold, making you a calorie-rich consumer. Therefore, the lactate threshold is a measure of your speed and the rate of fat loss. Professional athletes with a high lactate thresholds can be faster runners as well as burn more calories. This can increase their overall fitness.

Road racing is thus a great option for people who wish to increase their speed, lose weight and get fit, among other general health issues.

Track racing

Track racing is a different bike training program. If you're looking to be able to run quickly, you must be fast. That is the purpose of track racing. about. Track racing is a low-intensity interval training, but it will really increase your speed and endurance.

It is about going out for an extended distance ride, and then slotting into intervals, and then recovering intervals. Researchers from MacMaster University found out that this is a good way to recover intervals, particularly for those exercising at a high intensity and need to relax.

It's effect is improving your cardiovascular system. A stronger cardiovascular system ensures that your body is supplied with oxygen rich blood. Muscles become more efficient in utilising oxygenated blood. It is when your nervous system as well as the muscles gets supercharged and results in increased speed of rotation. Speed increases too.

On the track, you should start by running an estimated 300m in 80 percent your speed. You should include a two or three minutes of recovery, where you have the option of going slower or just rest for a while. Increase these distances to ensure that you recover carefully.

When you are an expert, you must start by running impressive distances.

Mountain Biking

It involves riding off the main roads, mostly on bumpy terrain. Some people prefer specially designed bicycles for this kind of workout. Contrary to the two training programs we've discussed previously mountain bike riding is intense training regimen.

The best part about the program is that it doesn't don't require a lot of time. A mere just 10 minutes will be sufficient to push you over the edge!

The sport of mountain biking is shown to be extremely fast and efficient method to speed up. It boosts the VOX2Max i.e. it boosts the oxygen consumption of your body to its highest levels. You've probably heard people claim that those who live in hills are better athletes. However, nothing could be further from the fact. Increased VOX2Max significantly increases the speed of your run and boosts your energy levels.

Mountain biking begins with the identification of your preferred trail. It is recommended to set up sprints in certain parts of the trail as well as places that are flat to recover from the workout. Repetition the hill climbs at regular intervals to achieve the best outcomes. Your training should be long and rigorous to test your abilities and endurance.

Training on stationary bikes

Stationery bikes are an easy method to exercise. They are advantageous in that you are able to be watching TV while engaging in your workouts. But, you'll need to have to be disciplined for this to be effective. I recommend that you set goals you want to achieve during your exercise prior to the workout.

Do some off-the-saddle hill climbs that incorporates high resistance, low number of revolutions per minute, and sitting in the pedals. This could cause a reaction on your hamstrings as well as muscles. Change to sprints that have lower resistance while keeping your speed of revolutions per minute as high as feasible. Certain cruising may require to use low resistance, and slow speeds.

If you are able to complete at least 30 minutes exercise every days of your week it will definitely benefit you. I know of a few great athletes who can do it for more than 2 hours. But, you shouldn't make the decision to add more time to your routine workouts abruptly. The length of training must be gradual in order to prevent potential injuries. If you are looking to recuperate take advantage of short rides into your stationery bike, allowing your body to recuperate.

Chapter 9: Running Hiit Running

Time: 15 minutes

Force: MODERATE to HARD

Timed/Reps: TimED

Planes of Motion: SAGITTAL, FRONTAL, and TRANSVERSE

Tone that include ABS, WAIST CORE, LEGS, and BOTTOM

RPE 5-7

Enhance your running endurance and speed by doing this HIIT exercise. The shorter bursts of greater intensity will boost your speed and boost your stamina for running. When you are done with the workout, it is advised to perform 20 power blasts side-to-side as this is an effective plyometric movement that helps build strength in your legs as well as bring in the extra direction of motion. As you become more fit and stronger, you can incorporate the 15-minute program that is provided alongside your running. Making use of slight grades as slopes are a great way to develop power in your lower body, which in the last , helps increase the speed you run.

THE 15-MINUTE ROUTINE

Two minutes, 30 second running at a standard pace 5 levels

20 seconds run as quick as possible: Level 7

10 seconds delicate running: Level 5

Rehash 5 times

Finalize with 40 POWER SIDE TO SIDE BLASTS

Running TIP

Inhale through your mouth and nose to ensure that you receive plenty of oxygen into your muscle during running. If you are running at a slower pace, you should be breathing deeply in the midsection as it will counteract any edges.

The FREE WEIGHTS HIIT WORKOUT

Time: 15 minutes

Energy: MODERATE to HARD

Reps and Coordinated: Timing and Reps

Planes of Motion: SAGITTAL and TRANSVERSE

Tone: BICEPS, SHOULDERS, TRICEPS, OBLIQUES, LEGS, BOTTOM, and ABS

RPE 5 to 7.5

This workout shows that HIIT doesn't have to be about exercise! It is possible to achieve amazing results through a combination of free weights and cardio, and the benefit of both methods of training is that both are fat-burners that are high in calories. Combining them creates an energised, solid body and also allows you to the body to shed excess fat by boosting your metabolic rate at rest (the quantity of calories that your body consumes). It stays elevated for an extended time following your exercise. Prior to starting your workout, make sure you have completed your warm-up. If you are using exercises that are free, I suggest that you use a weight you are able to lift 8 to 12 repetitions prior to feeling challenging, and a good method is to find the weight that is hitting that point of challenge. In the event that you feel shaky after a few reps you feel the weight is not large, and if think you are able to prop it the weight up for 25 reps then the weight is too thin.

1. EXERCISE HIGH KNEES ON PLACE

While running in place, try to raise your knees by squeezing through your arms. Maintain your back straight and slowly land. Repeat this exercise for 60 seconds, and then slowly move in place for 10 seconds.

EXERCISE 2: ALTERNATE BICEP CURLS

Keep your body straight and your arms folded so that two weights are on your chest. Slowly begin to lower one weight to your hip. Your arm is being straightened. When you are done, raise the weight again then switch the arms. Keep alternating for 20 repetitions.

Exercise 3: HIGH KNEES in PLACE

In a steady pace, you should try to raise your knees and then siphoning them through your arms. Maintain your back straight and then land gently. Perform this for about 50 seconds, and afterwards, slowly move into the same direction for 10 seconds.

4th EXERCISE: WEIGHTED SIDE BENDS

Place your free weights on the opposite one side. Slowly curve your body to the opposite side, and bring the weight to your knee, while keeping the weight that is hidden from sight. Take a second to hold then slowly lower the weight back to your knee, moving between sides. Your knees must remain soft and your abdominal muscles tucked in. Do not lean back or forward. Make sure you complete 22 repetitions.

Exercise 5: HIGH KNEES IN PLACE

While running in place, try to lift your knees by squeezing them with your arms. Maintain your back straight, and then land gently. Repeat this for 40 seconds. Then, afterwards, gently move into your position for 10 seconds.

Exercise 6: Weighted SQUAT

Maintain a straight posture with good posture and your arms by your sides. Hold on to your weights. Slowly twist and then enter an squat. Make an effort to keep the weights as close to the floor as you are able and then push them back up. Try to complete 20 repetitions.

EXERCISE 7 HIGH KNEES in PLACE

While running in place, try to raise your knees by squeezing them with your arms. Maintain your back straight and then land gently. Perform it for 30 minutes. Then afterwards, gently move in place for 10 seconds.

EXERCISE 8 AFRAID WEIGHT LUNGE

Maintain a good posture, keeping the arms are between your thighs. Now, push forward onto your left leg, while at the same time bringing both your arms towards your chest.

Maintain this position and then lower the left leg and then climb up and stand, then straighten your arms. When you are standing, jump on the right footand play in a biceps turn using the weights. Mean to do 20 exchanging repetitions.

EXERCISE 9 HIGH NOSE PRESENT

In a steady pace, you should try to raise your knees by squeezing them with your arms. Maintain your back straight, and then land gently. Repeat this for 20 minutes and afterwards, gently move in place for 10 seconds.

Exercise 10: FREE WEIGHT CHEST

Reclining on the ground, you can hold the weights you have free of hands bowed, and your arms looking towards the future. Now, gradually raise the two arms up to the top of you. Hold them for a few seconds, then slowly lower the weights. Try to complete 20 reps. Take a 30 second rest time, drink some water, then repeat the exercise. Then, finish with some chill-off stretch.

The HIIT SKIPPING Workout

Time: Under 8 minutes

Power: Power:

Coordinated/Reps: Timed and Reps

Plans of Movement: SAGITTAL, FRONTAL, and TRANSVERSE

Tone that include: CHEST, LEGS BACK, ARMS, and ABS

RPE 6 to 7.5

For this intense exercise the only thing you'll need is an exercise jump rope. This workout consists of skipping movements that are high-force, joined by three movements that make use of the jump rope with no skipping! I designed this workout so that you will get a fantastic cardiovascular workout, as well as a remarkable muscle training with my intriguing non-skip exercises. Begin your warm-up.

EXERCISE 1 LEFT LEG HOP KIP

You can skip by performing a jumping skipping on your left leg for 30 minutes. If you're not familiar with skipping, you should stick to a basic skip.

EXERCISE 2 SQUAT JUMP ROPE

The skipping rope should be laid on the floor and stand close to it. Squat down and then jump over the rope getting into a deep squat. After that, you can jump across the rope. Perform 30 repetitions.

EXERCISE 3: DOUBLE-FEET SKIP

Jump two feet above the ground at the same time. Try to leap high, and then land gently. Try this for 30 seconds.

4. EXERCISE 4. HORIZONTAL AB JUMP

Set the jump rope down in the middle of the flooring. Take a step onto the floor with your feet and hands. Put your hands on the opposite end of the other side of the rope. Place your feet on the opposite end of the rope. You can jump them high, then place your feet on the other edge of rope. Rehash for 30 times.

Exercise 5: RIGHT LEG HOP SKIP

Perform skipping bounces with the right foot. You should do this for 30 minutes. If you're new to skipping, keep to a simple skip.

EXERCISE 6: the ultimate AB MOVE

Falsehood recumbent and legs expanded and a jump rope folded over feet. Take the two pieces of the bargains, then fold between your fingers until the rope is at an abrasion. Now, lift your shoulders and head off the floor and then dismantle the rope by moving it from side to side while keeping your shoulders and your head away from the floor.

Perform 30 repetitions. Re-run the workout, but decrease each workout by 10 thus, knock off 10 minutes (or 10 reps). After that, repeat the exercise the routine, and again squeezing in additional 10 , or even 10 times. Then, play your tension and then extends.

The SKINNY JEANS IN 3 MOVES HIIT TRAINING

Time: Less than 7 mins

The Power Level: MODERATE to HARD

Coordinated/Reps: Timing and Reps

Plans of Movement: SAGITTAL, FRONTAL, and TRANSVERSE

Tone: HIPS LEGS WAIST, BOTTOM, and the OUTER and INNER THIGHS

RPE 5-7

There is nothing more satisfying than that has been smothered and etched when you don your favourite pair of slim jeans. The workout is just three movements that are designed to concentrate on the different zones that define a pleasing shape within your jeans. The benefit of the exercises is that I've created them in a way that they are what we call "compound exercises." They join a lot of muscles. This is also a way to burn off a lot of calories in one go. This exercise is guaranteed to leave you feeling amazing wearing those slim jeans. Before you begin, perform your warm-up.

EXERCISE 1 SKINNY JEAN JUMP

Stand up with a good posture. Start straight up, and after which you will to land, then you will jump straight up again. Then and landing on the ground, jump straight into a deep squat, trying to connect your fingers on the floor. Do this and then repeat for 20 times.

EXERCISE 2 SPRAY YOUR BOTTOM LIFT

Start in a light standing squat, with your arms twisting. Maintain this position, and then extend your arms upwards using your arms over your head and pushing one leg to the side behind your back. For a second, hold the position and then really crush the lower part of the lifted leg with your fingers. Then return to the starting position, and repeat on the opposite leg. Perform 40 times of these.

EXERCISE 3 JEAN CURTSY

While maintaining a healthy posture, hips separated and arms crossed, slowly slide to the opposite side by pulling one leg behind you and then twisting your knees while maintaining your chest straight. Continue to hold and, after that, return back to your starting position. Perform 20 repetitions on one leg, then perform another 20 repetitions on the opposite leg. If you're desperate to look gorgeous wearing your stylish jeans at this moment, you can repeat this routine a few times and then end with a tense feeling.

The CALORIE-BURNING CHAIR HIIT Workout

Time: Under 10 mins

Energy: MODERATE to HARD

Reps/Coordinators: TIMED and Reps

Plans of Movement: SAGITTAL, FRONTAL, and TRANSVERSE

Tone that include ABS, ARMS WAIST BOTTOM, LEGS and BUST INNER AND OUTER ThIGHS

RPE 5-7

The only thing you require to do this workout is a chair or solid surface. I suggest that you set the chair on the wall so that it is stable. The seven exercises are designed provide you with a complete body fitness exercise. Using the chair can help increase your calories consumed. In addition, you should always use an incredible range of improvement with every exercise that will result in amazing results. Before beginning, you should do your warm-up.

Exercise 1: STEP Up

Place your feet on the chair. Take a step up, ensuring that your two feet are set on the chair. remain for a second and then lower. Lead by using one leg, for 30 second, then follow using the right leg for another 30 minutes. Maintain a great posture and pull your tummy into.

EXERCISE 2 CALERIE RUN

In a downward direction, incline your chair until your hips are lowered and your hands are firmly seated onto the chairs. The chair should be placed against a wall so that it won't slide. You can copy the motion of running and bring your knee towards your chest. Make sure to maintain your back straight and straight while rotating legs. Repeat this exercise for 30 seconds.

3rd EXERCISE: CHAIR SQUAT

You should face your chair, and stay in a solid stance. As you progress, lower into a deep squat and plan to place both hands onto the chairs. For an additional second, and the next step is to slowly push into the starting position. Perform 30 times.

4. EXERCISE AB And ARM TONER

In a downward direction, you should lean towards your chair after which you can ensure it's securely in place and will not slide. Make sure your body is straight with your hips lowered and your abdominal muscles are pulled back. Slowly remove one hand from the chair, and then contact the shoulder of the opposite hand, hold then lower your hand. After that, raise the opposite hand, bringing it into contact with the shoulder on the opposite side, making sure that the tummy muscles are engaged. Perform 30 times in total.

Exercise 5. ULTIMATE THIGH TONER

Sitting side-by-side with your chair, put one of your legs on the chair, and following you've squatted, move into the squat position. Make sure that you don't allow the knee's line the chance to cross your toes. After that, do a lower squat and hold it for a moment, then following that, come back up. Do 20 repetitions on the same leg, before switching sides to perform the opposite leg.

Exercise 6: CHAIR AB Blast

False prostrate with two legs and feet lying across the seat. Reach upwards and, using two hands, reach the top in the seat. Make sure to keep it for a moment before dropping. When you are ready, try to grasp the other edge of the seat using two hands. When you reach this point lower, and then come back up to reach the middle, then at this point lower, and then stretch to the opposite edge of the chair. Complete 40 reiterations. Make sure that your tummy muscles are engaged.

Exercise 7 CHAIR LUNGE

Take a step away from the chair and place with one leg on your chair. Spread your arms ahead of you, making sure that your front foot is enough in the direction to ensure that, when you fall down your knee , it doesn't cross the line between the toes. Keep your abdominal muscles tight and your chest straight. Slowly lower yourself down to the floor then hold it for a moment, then the next time, push upwards.

Repeat this for 30 minutes on one leg before moving to the next. After you've completed this workout, make sure you do your chill-off stretches.

Foam Rolling Tips

Start with lighter rollers, and then increase the thickness. There are a variety of densities for froth and, if you're just starting out, you should leave the roller that is more gentle. Then you can move on to a more dense roller or even its awe-inspiring advanced version: the RumbleRoller (which includes the edges as well as torment grooves). While rolling each muscle, make it a goal to keep the fragile zones for 30 to one second. Take a deep breath and contemplate the muscle being unwinding as it can trigger an emotional response in the muscle that causes it to unwind. Our muscles are encased in connective tissue, also known as sash. It can grow and eventually become packed after a certain period of time. This may cause discomfort or irritation, and prompt us to pay back by altering the normal development patterns. Remuneration and development adjustments can cause injury. Thus, the froth roll can be an effective method to maintain the entire range of motion and protect our muscles from regular fitness and wellness workouts.

Do not roll over joints within your body, specifically your elbows, knees or your lower leg. Rolling is a way of paving the way for the joint, but it is never completed. Be cautious when you roll your back muscles to maintain your spine straight; refrain from bending between sides since we have ribs with gliding motions that are certainly not ones you would want to roll.

It is definitely not a separate method. Its benefits are comparable to tissue rubs, but this is the way to go that you are the specialist in back rub. That means you must perform a little bit of work by securing your body weight while you move. In the event that this puts stress upon your wrists lower into your lower arms, or reduce the amount of weight you put on your arms by shifting your arms as needed. The more you do this, the easier it'll become.

A Few HIIT Tips for beginners

*HIIT isn't recommended for people who are new to fitness or suffering from heart problems or knee, hip and joint phobias. Make sure to consult your primary physician prior to beginning any fitness program, and be mindful of your body. In conclusion that, there are various ways to incorporate the HIIT method in your initial fitness regimen, including an example of a few low-sway HIIT strategies:

It's not necessary to do a full-on workout. If you're a seasoned or moderately exerciser who has a good fitness regimen You'll be able to push yourself in interval sets. If you're just starting out, you should be able to quickly complete 30 minutes of uninterrupted exercise, every day week prior to exploring various ways to deal with speed increases. Beginners: If you go for 30 minutes to walk or run every day You are improving your cardiovascular fitness as well as improving your fitness level, and burning calories! Once you are satisfied with this, you may talk with your doctor about taking part in interval training.

*Look for shorter work periods and longer periods of rest. A great starting point is between 20 and 30 minutes of all the demanding exercise and 2 minutes of relaxation. Alternate between shorter exercises (10 up to fifteen minutes) before you start; increase the duration or reduce intervals until it is a lot easier). When you're comfortable using intervals or speed spikes, you may begin to expand the length of work, or decrease the length of rest.

*If you are looking for alternatives with low-sway, look into various options for joint-accommodating methods like cycling, curved, or swimming. The spin bike can be an excellent starting point to practice intervals. Many classes include beat exercises and speed drills that are great for increasing your heart rate while bringing it to a recovery state.

Running within the water is an additional excellent low-sway exercise option regardless of whether you're running by siphoning water or with submerged treadmills. Many rec centers provide water exercise classes which are easy on joints, particularly in the event that you've recently recovered from a sprain. If you're taking a water class be aware of an additional opposition from the water, and the faster and more intense the movements are, the more challenging it's going to be. Put your entire foot on the floor in the pool -- it very likely to entice "tippy-toe" throughout the entire time. You can also take note of the changes in the scenery! Similar to spin classes I didn't realize the level of difficulty water workouts might be until the point that I started to do them. I think it's similar to anything else that you get back the effort is put in it.

*For options for bodyweight cardio and plyometrics, beginners must remain on the ground for a long time. Do not bounce and try a small amount of movement. For example, during an squat then you'll reach for your floor (squat) and rise onto your feet with arms extended over your head. This can increase your heart rate , but without joint effects.

A simple method to make an activity easier and more difficult: slow down. I think that a lot people believe that speed is better, but maintaining a well-structured structure is a lot more crucial than speed. I'd prefer to see 10 great exercises that exceed 100 cringeworthy attempts to achieve a particular redundancy value. When you're trying to build a penance for speed, not just are you hitting the an entry point for injury, but you may also be depriving yourself into a more viable exercise. Focus on the muscles you're working when you're moving with a purpose through the exercise.

Integrating HIIT intervals into your daily routine

In order to help you make the most of your HIIT workouts, here's some ideas on how to integrate the workouts into your daily routine. There are a variety of options:

*HIIT and Strength. There are mixed opinions on whether it is better to finish the strength or cardio portion of your exercise first. My advice is to examine your goals and move from there. You'll likely have more energy for the main part of your workout and you can work more intensely. If fat-burning is your goal I suggest doing an HIIT or cardio part of your exercise first. If strengthening and building healthy muscles is your main goal, perform your strength workout first, then finish it off by doing cardio. At the end of the day the individual inclination will be vital. The combination doesn't make a huge difference going to the gym and working out will have a greater impact on your progress. The most effective workout is the one you'll perform.

*HIIT effects are interwoven with your strength training. The most effective strategy for HIIT is to complete a brief sequence of intervals of HIIT during your strength-building sets. This will increase your heart rate , and allow you to burn more calories throughout the workout as your heart rate is elevated during the tougher portions. (Likewise when you are circuit training, and then move quickly beginning with one exercise and moving to the next one, you will result in a more intense heart rate throughout your exercise.) In this method, do several sessions of strength workouts and add a cardio workout for 30 to 1 second before repeating the circuit of strength or moving towards the next series of exercises. (For example, if you're performing a circuit of pull-ups and squats as well as push-ups do the exercise for one set and include a few seconds of squat hops , and then repeat the circuit with squats, push-ups and pull-ups prior to doing squat hops again.)

*HIIT and the enduring state. This is among my favorite record-breaking HIIT methods. It is a method of performing HIIT intervals in any ratio (all fully explained in part 2.) And then, you'll combine it by performing simple state-of-the-art cardio. This will allow your body that it can effectively consume fat and allow your usual state exercises feel much easier. It's also amusing to add 5 minutes of high intensity intervals at the conclusion of a long time long run, or to mark the ultimate end of an unending, steady state-of-the-art cardio workout.

Common HIIT Errors

*Not making the rest of the interims too shorter or the work intermissions too long. As I mentioned previously Start small and gradually work upwards from there.

Perform HIIT workouts on days that are back-to-back. Allow your body to recuperate and rest by alternating the cardio force. Make sure you don't exercise at the same level that the previous day. My ideal seven-day workout comprises three days of intense exercise with two mild days and a simple day and an unplanned day.

Selecting exercises that don't bring your heart rate up within a short amount of time. I've seen HIIT recordings that use ordinary old biceps twists being used as "work" ratios. Most likely not. Choose something that is going to test your cardiovascular system quickly and you won't have to wait until you reach rep 12 to allow it to begin to work.

The role of recovery in the HIIT program.

Its very structure interferes with the normal resting state of the body, therefore recuperation is an integral part of any general workout routine. Recovery after exercise is crucial to the execution of the exercise, followed by improvement, and also a reduction in the risk of injury. This article focuses on the principles of recovery. It also describes how to use these guidelines to determine safe and effective recovery times for your workouts.

Many who exercise are inclined to have an tendency to focus on the workout, and not think about the events that occur prior or following. Exercisers spend much more of their time recuperating as opposed to an actual workout. If the speed of recovery is too short the higher volume of preparation and loads are impossible without the negative effects of excessive training. The time we dedicate to proper pre-and post-exercise recovery could be more crucial to improving execution and decrease damage than the exercise itself.

The high-power exercise specifically targets muscles and other tissues that are delicate and cause temporary destruction through tissues break down. A lack of recovery can reduce the transport of oxygen and supplements to the muscles working. This when combined with overtraining, reduces the ability to produce quality controlled, rapid, reduced maximal pulse, and a less resiliency to saw-effort rates. Recovery from physiological causes occurs mostly after exercise , and is defined by the physical efforts of the body's effort to get back to its equilibrium. The purpose behind exercising is to test homeostasis, or the body's normal internal balance.

Exercise disrupts the homeostasis process and, in turn, results in abnormalities at the compound sub-atomic, tissue, and levels. It is common for irritation to occur of the framework that is insusceptible to initiate a process that involves an increase in the flow of hormones, including cortisol and adrenaline to reduce the risk and speed up repair. The irritation and growth of muscles cause the process to go on. If the workout is too intense or long to the abilities and capabilities of the person exercising or the recovery is excessively brief or not allowed injuries and burnout could quickly occur.

The benefits of recovery

Recovery is crucial to achieve greater training volume and increases the ability to perform at higher levels without suffering negative effects of excessive training. Recovery helps to normalize the physiological capacity (e.g. returning blood pressure levels to pre-exercise levels, which then returns the body's breath to a resting state) also balances out the cardiovascular cycle and restores the pulse to normal levels. Recovery also restores the cell's condition back to be in a state of rest prior to exercise and plays a crucial role for the restoration of vitality, which includes muscle glycogen and blood glucose as well as other readily accessible energy sources that are essential for exercise. Recovery also triggers an adaptation response. As health improves, new muscle filaments and blood vessels grow and flourish and, in the end, interact with the structure of new neural pathways. A modified metabolic response allows higher levels of training and allows the body to adapt to the demands. Whatever the duration that the load is on it is possible for the body to become familiar with its new requirement to be able to effectively respond to increasing stresses.

In the words of the author, recovering from exercise could be more significant than the workout itself, since the repair and reconstruction of injured muscle tissue and the substitution of synthetic substances that are required can occur while recovering. A healthy recovery can limit the effects of physical stress training. The capacity to recover determines the ability to perform the next exercise. It is the source of the passion and mental energy needed to avoid fatigue as well as exhaustion and burnout.

Recovery Types

A healthy recovery is essential for all energy systems to function at its highest levels. The triphosphate adenosine (ATP) is the rapid source of energy needed for the compression of skeletal muscles however, it is limited by the intensity and length of the workout. Since ATP is essential for repeat muscles withdrawal, regardless of what energy system is being tasked with it and you can be sure that massive storage facilities of ATP are always available but this is not the case. Energy pathways are very different in the maximum amount of ATP depending on the length of time they are maintained. If you are performing anaerobic and amazing advancements, like the ones required by HIIT workouts included in this guide, the exhaustion begins to set in quickly. When training calls for both anaerobic pathways to produce ATP as well as intensity and time, these are the main factors in the creation of energy. Because high-intensity workouts tend to be repeated over various workouts as well as post-workout, recovery after the workout is an essential.

In-Workout Recovery

For HIIT programs, the intense period of recovery is referred to as the recovery in-workout as well as active recuperation. The recovery helps keep the body in motion and warm is a flow of dispersing waste products from exercise as well as allowing you to take a break and make a rational preparation to perform the next exercise. For example, in a tabata series you could do 20 seconds of work then rest and prepare for the next exercise session (the subsequent 20 second grouping) for a 10 second in-workout recovery phase. Recovery is essential since it eliminates acidosis and blood lactate levels during fast and hard workouts. This happens due to massive inhalations and exhalations as well as small changes in the body. The muscles function as siphons , which help to eliminate the body of waste products and to bring oxygen and nutrients back to the muscles that are working. The 10-second interval also aids in reducing heart rate, but it helps keep the heart moving to avoid blood accumulation in the smallest places and keep the heart rate to be above the minimal and below the most extreme to prepare for the next 20 second workout.

In HIIT protocols the duration of recovery of the ratio of training is usually negative, which means that the work session will be longer than the recuperation. For example when you are in the Tabata convention the ratio of training is 2:1, which means that the duration of the interval is double the duration of recovery (e.g. the work duration of 20 seconds, and an interval recovery of 10-seconds). The goal is to test the body's anaerobic resources, thereby challenging Type II filaments of muscle (quick jerk) which results in the development of oxygen debt as well as the longer-term abundance after exercise oxygen use (EPOC). The feeling of being exhausted is an important element of HIIT since it's a physiological sign that the workout is a high-intensity exercise and that your body may be in a state of oxygen debt.

In any event, HIIT conventions don't generally require negative recovery sessions. Certain HIIT techniques employ constructive recovery for example people who are incapable of performing exercises that utilize negative recovery. The most amazing aspect of HIIT is that ratios can be altered to deal with specific problems. It is crucial to note that regardless of the ratio used the consistency of use is crucial. For example, if you're employing a 1:2 ratio ensure that you adhere to the ratio. For instance, if your workout lasts 15 seconds, then the recovery phase should be 30 minutes. The ratio that is constant during a particular exercise will result in the physiological effects of breathlessness and ultimately EPOC an endocrine process that keeps the body taking in vitality while it repairs itself.

Chronic Recovery

Chronic recovery refers to the length of time that the body needs to recover after a HIIT exercise. Think of it as the period between workouts during the day and the next day in a certain week. Additionally, there are two kinds of chronic recovery: active and passive.

Active Recovery

Active recovery could be described as a moderate-to-direct power workout in between HIIT sessions. Since HIIT workouts are extremely demanding, taking an interested in an recovery exercise following a hard exercise (back in-back HIIT training sessions aren't recommended) will allow you to continue with an incredible preparation without risking your body due to uncontrollable burdens as well as overtraining, which can lead to the potential for injury to increase. The kind and strength of an active recovery depends on your own determination, but ruleslike and the associated guidelines can aid.

Allow adequate time between workouts

In all instances, allow for a period of 24 hours between workouts. They are not designed to be done in tandem. For example, if you do the HIIT exercise on Monday, do the same exercise on Wednesday or Thursday , to ensure that you have enough recovery.

Do not neglect recovery Between Exercises

The recovery workouts don't burden the vitality and anaerobic frameworks as HIIT training does; Instead, they boost the healing process and repair damaged tissues to produce faster and more powerful units. Training at moderate intensity for less than 75 minutes will decrease general aggravation and improve positive synapses (for instance, serotonin or endorphins) and stimulate the development of animate nerves and increase the flow of blood to those working on the muscles, as well as to the cerebrum. For example, if you completed a 30- to 45 minutes of HIIT on Monday, the following Tuesday, you should engage in an activity that requires oxygen (pulse exercise at 5 , 6, or 7 on a range of 1 to 10 such as supine cycling or a circular exercise and strolling on a treadmill or outdoors or in an Pilates or yoga workout that focuses on quality stability, and adaptability instead of intense work. In the course of your training for the long term by focusing on equilibrium (high-power exercises, high-exertion ones that are separated by low-force workouts) can provide you with the best results, without risking injuries from abuse, inadequate recovery as well as, at the end, burning out.

Start preparing to begin the transition and transition out

Warm-up regularly and chill off prior to beginning any exercise which includes detached and dynamic exercises for recovery. Consider the stress placed on your car while you're sitting and then suddenly increase speed to 60 miles per hour (97 kilometers per hour) in just a few minutes. It's similar to what your body experiences when you do not engage in an appropriate warm-up prior to exercising. Because the purpose of the purpose of warming up is to set the body up for future exercises, it is important to think of it not unlike a physiological preparation. The workouts and exercises you choose for your warm-up must be guided by the task you're planning to perform. The warm-up should be enough to boost the central body temperature, increase the temperature of joints (e.g. hips, knees, shoulders spine segment) boost blood flow to major muscles, and raise sweat.

The chill that is gone or the transition from exerciseshould allow you to transition from activity to rest, with the least amount of sacrifice. Have you ever gone to shower after exercise and found you're not yet sweating? This indicates that the transition from exercise was insufficient to bring your pulse closer to resting levels, reduce blood flow to the muscles working and to make sure that your body knows that the workout part of the day has been completed. The break between exercise and transition is also an excellent moment to make use of warm muscles through the static or, if held stretching. Because the muscles are flexible and warm and flexible, they are likely to react to held stretch. It is also important to put aside the effort to return your body to a slumbering state.

Sleep Enough

Sleep is an essential recovering device. The right amount of sleep allows the body to recover and repair itself during exercise. Research suggests that between 7 and 9 hours of rest every night is the most important factor to maintain hormonal balance and physical recovery. Sleep enhances the effects of muscle building of exercise through a broader the protein mix, and helps the nervous system return to a state of relaxation. Sleep boosts the capacity to resist which aids in the healing of muscle tissue as well as metabolism balance.

Signs of overtraining

Particularly when using the plyometric (hopping and explosive) exercises as part or HIIT exercises, it's always advisable to be aware of the signs of excessive training. Overtraining is a problem set aside by the inability to properly recover between workouts exercising too vigorously and completing excessive training sessions each week, or failing to follow suggested recovery and training proportions and guidelines.

Overtraining is essential in the beginning of the program and when you put the exercise on hold in the aftermath of illness or injury. Training levels and decreases in performance as well as injuries and burnout are clear indications of excessive training. If at the very least one of the accompanying signs or indicators are present, the power of training and duration, recurrence, or duration must be decreased until they disappear.

* Unable to finish an effective training session

* An increasing amount of inflammation of the muscles that starts after a training session, and then to the next

* Excessive muscle discomfort and firmness after a workout

* A sudden diminishing in body weight

* Insomnia

* Injuries to joints or stress cracks discomfort

* A growth in the resting pulse

Passive Recovery

Passive recovery is considered in two distinct methods: (1) recovery that is swiftly triggered after an anaerobic workout or (2) more prolonged passive exercises that happen during high-force training sessions. In the first instance it is a quick recovery after an HIIT interlude to replenish ATP-CP storage and to eliminate the waste products that build up as a result of the high-force activities. The replenishment and recovery for these frameworks is crucial because they perform an important role in the production of vitality after-effects of a high-power interval. Passive recovery could involve simply lying down or laying down after an exercise session.

The problem with the inability to recover quickly after an exercise session is that waste productslike lactic corrosive, lactic acid and other concoction ingredients are slow to disappear when recovering dynamically, and blood could accumulate in the lower body. The most preferred approach is that ATP-CP resynthesis becomes increasingly rapid; in addition the fact that the longer the time to recover and the greater replenishment occurs. In the Tabata standard, recovery is only 10 seconds and, in this case it is recommended that you don't rest or sit between workouts, in order to use the muscles as siphons to avoid blood pooling at your areas. Maintaining a healthy lifestyle also considers a rapid elimination of waste products , as well as replenishment of ATP-CP. This assists in removing waste and stimulates the system.

Different strategies are useful to help you recover passively between workouts for the body to return to a state of rest. This section focuses on the usage the foam roller to aid in active recovery in after HIIT exercises.

Foam rollers are a useful piece of exercise hardware. The self-massage process is known as self-myofascial release or SMR. The foam roller can be used to get to the tissues in the area that the belt (the the encasement of muscles) and the ligaments and the muscles and tendons. Rolling may aid in unwinding muscles, releasing knots and bonds, removing the waste materials, and generally improving circulation and blood circulation.

Rollers are available in a variety in sizes, densities and shapes. The harder, thinner rollers are significantly more impressive than softer, less dense models. The typical roller is 3 feet (90 centimeters) long and six inches (15 centimeters) wide. Some rollers come with tracks that can increase the power in the process. The following are the general guidelines for self-massage using the foam roller:

* Roll between 2 and 3 inches (5 to 8 cm) at a time, avoiding from rolling on joints as well as bones.

* Slowly roll, maintaining control over the lower back and bears.

* Make sure you maintain a great posture while rolling, drawing the center and settling your spine.

* If an attachment or knot is felt while rolling, try to eliminate it by putting your body at that location for a few seconds. A slight discomfort is not be unusual, nevertheless, there is there should be no discomfort. If the knot doesn't ease within a short time then move on and return to the same area at a later moment, perhaps over the course of a few days.

* If you experience pain, quit rolling. Rolling when the pain is present can increase discomfort and cause pain. Damage could result.

* Resting for 20-30 minutes on the painful area can help to energize unwinding and reduce tension and discomfort.

* You are able to roll a few times during the day, for whatever amount of time you're comfortable with.